INFLUENZA: THE LAST GREAT PLAGUE

An unfinished story of discovery

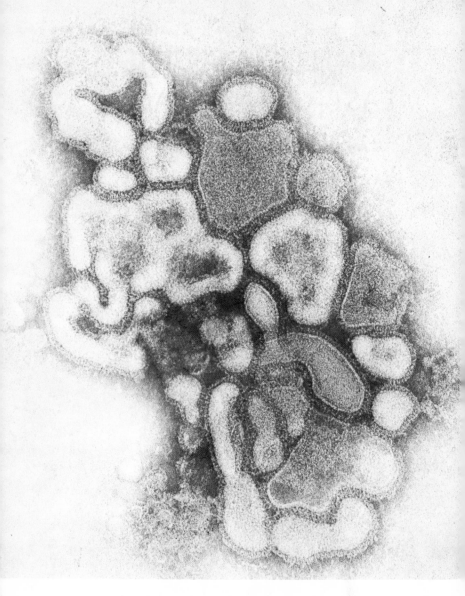

Specimen Influenza A/NJ/8/76 (Hsw1 N1)
Magnification 132,000; Date: 2-20-76
Courtesy *Center for Disease Control*

INFLUENZA: THE
LAST GREAT PLAGUE

An unfinished story of discovery

W. I. B. BEVERIDGE

PRODIST
New York
1977

First published in the United States by
PRODIST
a division of
Neale Watson Academic Publications, Inc.
156 Fifth Avenue, New York, New York 10010

Library of Congress Cataloging in Publication Data

Beveridge, William Ian Beardmore, 1908–
   Influenza : the last great plague.

   Includes index.
   1. Influenza. 2. Epidemiology. I. Title.
RC150.B4 1977   614.5'18   77-2971
ISBN 0-88202-118-4

Manufactured in the U.S.A.

Contents

v

Foreword

by **Sir Christopher Andrewes,** *formerly Director of the World Influenza Centre, London*

Influenza is something unique. It behaves epidemiologically in a way different from that of any other known infection. We have learnt in recent years that the influenza A virus infects a variety of birds and mammals besides man. Professor Beveridge has written an informative account of the infection and, having a background in veterinary medicine, has given due weight to 'flu infections of animals generally. His book is of particular value in two ways. His learned account of the history of the disease contains much that will be unfamiliar even to workers in the field; this all helps to put the disease into perspective. Then he discusses fully modern ideas of the part which 'animal' influenzas may play in the strange epidemiology of influenza. Current research should soon reveal to us just what is going on. We must hope that the knowledge gained will help us control the disease and thwart the virus' unpleasant habit of effecting, every decade or so, a protean change, which enables it to start up a fresh pandemic.

Preface

Pestilences of many sorts have brought death and misery to mankind throughout history. Over the last 100 years most of these plagues have been brought under control; the black death, cholera, yellow fever, typhus, and smallpox no longer rage unchecked every few years. But there is one disease that continues to flourish and cause pandemics that sweep around the world periodically without restraint by modern medical science: the last of the great plagues is influenza.

Until the last few years the origin of these worldwide epidemics – called pandemics – was a mystery. At long last we have a theory of how they arise. In language the non-medical reader can understand this book describes how investigators in many countries have followed clues and gradually accumulated knowledge that enables us to understand the natural history of the minute organism that has killed millions of people – 20 millions in one pandemic – and is one of the greatest enemies of man. We still do not know enough to be able to prevent pandemics, but the quest has reached the exciting stage where we think we know the stronghold of the enemy, the biological home of the virus. Surprisingly, the evidence suggests that the primitive breeding ground of influenza viruses is in wild birds. But the interrelationship of viruses found in man with those found in birds and mammals is a complicated one; it is not a simple matter of influenza spreading from animals to man. The virus must undergo subtle changes before it can infect man.

Some of the worst plagues of man are caused by microbes whose biological home is in animals. The black death (bubonic and pneumonic plague) which periodically killed off a large percentage of the population in medieval times is caused by a microbe that lives in rats. Yellow fever, which used to kill innumerable people in tropical and subtropical countries and long delayed the construction of the Panama canal, is a disease of monkeys. It used to be thought that influenza spread from horses and other animals to man, but since the beginning of this century it has been regarded as primarily, if not exclusively, a human disease. Only during the last few years has evidence been uncovered that has changed our whole concept of the natural history of this remarkable and unique virus.

It has been my good fortune to be able to follow closely the unfolding of this story of discovery over the last forty years and to know personally the enthusiasts who have led the investigations. It makes a fascinating tale with all the puzzlement and excitement of a detective novel. My purpose in writing this book is twofold: to interest and enlighten the general reader, and to provide the doctor, research virologist, and public health authority with a panoramic view of the epidemic behaviour of influenza from the earliest historical records to the latest research. Our knowledge seems to me to have reached a stage where we need to review the whole situation and plan the future strategy against this resourceful enemy. I believe it is time to start looking for ways of preventing pandemics.

I am very grateful to the following colleagues who read the typescript and offered helpful criticism: Sir Christopher Andrewes, Professor Leslie Banks, Dr Konrad Bögel, Dr Paul Brès, Dr Martin Kaplan, and Dr Geoffrey Schild. Dr H. P. Chu, Dr Bernard Easterday, and Dr Robert Webster have kindly allowed me to mention some of their research results which have not yet been published. My special thanks are due to Miss Margaret McKean for her endless patience and care with typing the manuscript and helping with references.

The views on the ecology of influenza virus expounded in this book were first outlined by me in *Frontiers in Comparative Medicine* published by the University of Minnesota Press in 1972. Finally I wish to express my appreciation for the excellent co-operation that I have enjoyed with Heinemann Educational Books Ltd.

1976   W.I.B.B.

1

How the cause was discovered

At one time it was thought that influenza epidemics were due to the malevolent influence of heavenly bodies such as planets, comets, and meteors. At other times the disease was attributed to volcanic eruptions and earthquakes that were believed to allow poisonous gases to escape from the earth. Sometimes the weather was blamed. But along with these fanciful notions about the origin of the epidemics there was a vague idea that the spread of the disease was in some way due to the dissemination of a mysterious malign agent, called a miasma, that is a condition of the air something like a bad smell.

There is a good description of the 1793 influenza epidemic in Philadelphia by Robert Johnson writing in 1806. He postulated that the disease was propagated at least to some extent by contagion, but the editor of Johnson's publication added a footnote saying he disagreed, as he believed the disease to be '*exclusively* of atmospheric origin . . . probably a deleterious gas'. It is in fact less than a century since the contagious nature of many diseases has been generally accepted. As recently as 1894 the eminent British epidemiologist Charles

Creighton did not believe influenza was spread by contagion. He cited medical opinion during the epidemics of 1833, 1837, and 1847, when the doctrine of contagiousness was out of favour because the disease affected most parts of the country in the same two or three weeks, affected the population within a considerable radius almost at once and the occupants of a house simultaneously. It was argued that these are not the marks of disease that pass from one person to another. Creighton preferred the concept of a miasma spreading over the land.

However, Creighton's views were by no means generally held at the time of the 1889–90 pandemic, as most doctors had by then accepted the germ theory of infectious diseases. Research workers concentrated on trying to find a bacterial cause and in Germany Richard Pfeiffer discovered a particular bacterium present in great numbers in the throats of patients with influenza. It was called 'Pfeiffer's influenza bacillus', but not everyone was convinced that it was the cause of the disease.

In 1918 came the great pandemic of Spanish influenza that caused dreadful mortality and tremendous social and economic disruption. This had the effect of stimulating intensive research into the cause of the disease. Bacteriologists again found large numbers of Pfeiffer's bacillus in patients' throats. Attempts were made to determine whether it really was the cause of influenza by placing drops of cultures in the noses of volunteers. Usually these inoculations had no effect, although in a few instances it was claimed that influenza had been produced.

By 1918 it was known that some diseases are caused by microbes smaller than bacteria. They were referred to as 'filtrable viruses' because they could pass through filters that held back bacteria, or 'ultra-visible' viruses because they could not be seen with the ordinary microscope. These are what we now call viruses. So experiments were undertaken to ascertain whether the cause of Spanish influenza was a virus, but the technical methods then available were crude. Monkeys, rabbits, and other animals were inoculated with throat washings from patients, some having been passed through filters to hold back bacteria, but the results were mostly negative. A few animals developed mild symptoms that were considered not significant. In a rather heroic effort, a series of inoculation experiments was carried out in human volunteers. At first some successful transmissions were claimed when filtered sputum and juices from the lungs of fatal cases were used, but in the great majority of experiments no illness was produced and the general conclusion was that the experiments did not support the 'filter passer' hypothesis. The net result of these extensive investigations was to increase the bewilderment and to deepen the mystery. Robert Donaldson of St George's Hospital Medical School, London, wrote in 1922 'there is not the slightest shred of evidence that the disease is due to a so-called filter-passing virus'* and in 1929, W. M. Scott of the British Ministry of Health wrote 'there is little hope that they [the difficulties] will ever be overcome in the case of influenza'†. It is interesting and salutary to read, in the light of present day knowledge, these text-books written in the 1920s. They contain a curious mixture of obscure

---

* Robert Donaldson, in *Influenza*, ed. F. G. Crookshank, (London: William Heinemann, 1922).

† W. M. Scott. *A System of Bacteriology*, Med. Res. Council Vol. II., (London: H. M. Stationery Office, 1929).

reasoning and jargon not so very different in character from what one reads now about those aspects of influenza we still do not understand.

SWINE INFLUENZA

The cause of influenza was discovered not by a direct attack on the human disease but in a round about way from studies on an animal disease. In other words, comparative medicine provided the key discovery that led to the solution of this mystery, as it has with so many others in human medicine. In passing it may be pointed out that all types of pathogenic microbes – fungi, protozoa, bacteria, mycoplasma, and viruses – were first found to be the cause of diseases in animals and only subsequently were they shown to cause disease in man.

An astute veterinarian, J. S. Koen of Fort Dodge, Iowa, working as an inspector of the U.S.A. Bureau of Animal Industry, observed a disease in pigs which he believed was the same disease as Spanish influenza. Koen's views were not popular with pig farmers as they feared that consumers would be put off eating pork. But Koen had the courage and conviction to stick to his guns against both opposition and scepticism and insisted that the disease in pigs was a new one which arose during the second wave of the 1918 pandemic. Here is Koen's defence of his diagnosis, written in 1919:

> 'Last fall and winter we were confronted with a new condition, if not a new disease. I believe I have as much to support this diagnosis in pigs as the physicians have to support a similar diagnosis in man. The similarity of the epidemic among people and the epidemic among pigs was so close, the reports so frequent, that an outbreak in the family would be followed immediately by an outbreak among the hogs, and *vice versa*, as to present a most striking coincidence if not suggesting a

close relation between the two conditions. It looked like "flu", and until proved it was not "flu", I shall stand by that diagnosis.'

In 1928, veterinarians in the Bureau of Animal Industry led by C. N. McBryde successfully transmitted influenza from pig to pig by taking mucus from the respiratory tract of sick pigs and instilling it into the noses of healthy pigs. However they failed in their attempts to transmit the disease by inoculating material that had been filtered. The types of bacterial filter then available were crude by present day standards and probably little or no virus got through the filters used.

About this time a brilliant young medical graduate, Richard Shope, was working at the Rockefeller Institute for Comparative Pathology at Princeton, New Jersey, which was under the directorship of the renowned Theobald Smith. The concept to which this Institute was dedicated was that many of the basic phenomena of disease can best be studied in animals and plants. Shope was an extrovert and unconventional thinker receptive to novel ideas. He was intrigued by Koen's observations and visited pig farmers in the Midwest where he found that swine influenza still occurred every autumn. In the autumn of 1928 he repeated McBryde's experiments using the excellent facilities available at the Institute at Princeton. By inoculating unfiltered material Shope reproduced the disease under strict experimental conditions. More importantly, pigs also became ill when he used filtered fluid for inoculation. The disease produced by the filtrate was mild but it could be transferred repeatedly in pigs. This can be taken as the first reliable experimental evidence that influenza is caused by a virus and it provided the basis for further research along these lines into influenza in man.

I.—2

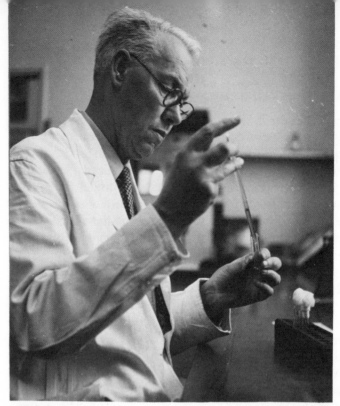

Christopher Andrewes, one of the team that isolated the first human influenza virus in 1933, and the first director of the World Influenza Centre, London. (Photo by courtesy WHO.)

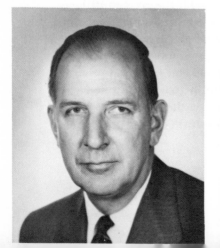

Richard Shope who isolated influenza virus from swine in 1931, before it had been demonstrated in man. (Photo by courtesy Rockefeller University.)

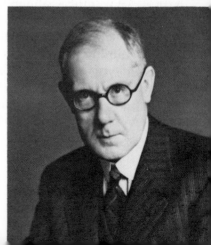

Wilson Smith, one of the team who isolated the first influenza virus from man in 1933; he was the first to cultivate the virus in chick embryos in 1935. (Photo Walter Stoneman

THE FIRST HUMAN INFLUENZA VIRUS

Shope's research was published in 1931. In January 1933, an epidemic of human influenza occurred in England and Christopher Andrewes and Wilson Smith, who were working on viruses at the National Institute for Medical Research, London, were asked to make another attempt at finding the cause. Influenza in man was still regarded as a mystery but in the light of Shope's work it was thought worth while attempting to demonstrate its viral cause by inoculating filtrates of human throat washings into various animals. At first Andrewes and Wilson Smith made injections into various parts of the body of the animals, neglecting to drop the inoculum into the nose as McBryde and Shope had done and which we now know is the only route by which influenza can be transmitted.

While these experiments were being carried out, Wilson Smith was told of an epidemic of influenza in the staff of the Wellcome Laboratories, London. What was of special interest was that ferrets kept there for research on canine distemper had also become ill, seemingly from influenza. So Wilson Smith inoculated some ferrets with filtrates and this time he dropped the fluid into their noses, remembering the Americans' technique with pigs. Meanwhile Andrewes had himself fallen ill with influenza and it was the washings from his throat that Wilson Smith filtered and inoculated into the ferrets. The day that Andrewes returned to work the ferrets showed clear signs of respiratory disease – sneezing, discharge from nose and eyes, and raised temperature. At long last a virus had been demonstrated in a case of influenza in man. However, by a curious irony, the disease in ferrets at the Wellcome Laboratories turned out not to be influenza after all, but canine distemper! It has truly been said that an hypothesis can be useful even if it is not correct.

The early work was by no means plain sailing and there were many false trails and snags to be overcome before the technique of transmitting the virus consistently from ferret to ferret by filtrates was worked out. Then another lucky break came. While one of the scientists was examining an inoculated ferret it sneezed in his face and a couple of days later he sickened with influenza. This was just what was needed to confirm that the virus isolated in ferrets was indeed the human influenza virus.

Shope then tried inoculating ferrets with his swine influenza virus. Now, ferrets are awkward animals to handle and Shope found they struggled violently when he attempted to put drops in their noses, and were inclined to sneeze the fluid back at him. You will remember that Shope believed the virus he was handling was the one that caused the severe 1918 influenza, and he did not like the idea of having it sneezed back into his face. Therefore he anaesthetized the ferrets before inoculating them. He found that ferrets treated in this way not only developed a fever and runny nose but also pneumonia, as is sometimes seen in man. As soon as Andrewes and Wilson Smith heard of this they tried it on ferrets with their human virus and found it worked equally well. Then they decided to try inoculating mice again, with which they had previously had no results, but this time under anaesthetic. The mice took the disease and developed pneumonia and large doses killed them. It was then realized that fluid dropped into the noses of animals when they were anaesthetized gets down into their lungs. At last here was a relatively simple and inexpensive technical method for experimenting with influenza virus and from then on influenza research moved swiftly.

In 1935, Wilson Smith discovered that influenza virus can be cultivated by inoculating it into a developing chick embryo. (Fertile hens eggs, that have been incubated for ten days, are inoculated with virus. After two days further incubation one can harvest several millilitres of fluid that contains up to 10 000 million virus particles and comparatively little extraneous protein.) Soon afterwards it was found that the virus caused red blood cells to clump together and that the antibody against the virus prevented the clumping. These simple techniques made influenza virus one of the easiest viruses to work with in the laboratory, so many virologists all over the world were attracted to influenza research. Consequently we now know more about this virus than almost any other affecting man.

One of the first things learnt was that there are three types of the virus all of which have the same appearance under the electron microscope but have no relationship whatever to each other so far as immunity to them is concerned. The types are called A, B, and C. Type A is by far the most important and most interesting and so far as we know is the only one that causes serious pandemics and the only one that occurs naturally in animals. Type B gives rise to epidemics, though less frequently than A and often they are confined mainly to children of school age. Type C is uncommon and unimportant and may be entirely left out of our discussion.

The next discovery was that type A strains are not all identical although they are related. When the relationship is distant they are said to belong to different *subtypes*, when the relationship is close but they are not exactly the same, they are said to be *variants*. The degree of relationship is estimated by the extent to which a vaccine made from one virus will immunize an animal against a second virus. If the cross immunity is strong, the viruses are judged to be identical; if it is weak, the viruses are said to be related and the degree of the relationship is measured by the extent of protection when quantitative experiments are done. The whole question of interrelationships of influenza viruses will be explained in Chapter 6.

This chapter should serve to introduce the general reader to the subject. I shall now go on to describe the disease, its history and its epidemic behaviour in man and animals. The reader will then have an understanding of the problem that faces the research worker and will be able to appreciate the significance of the research as the story unfolds in the subsequent chapters. Finally I shall suggest some fields for research that I believe should now be pursued urgently.

2

The disease in the individual and in the population

Today it is often said that a person has influenza when he really has only a severe common cold, and consequently the seriousness of the disease this book is about tends to be underrated in the public's estimation. The description of the disease and its history in this and the next chapter show that true influenza ranks among the great plagues of mankind.

First let us consider the illness as it affects the individual. The incubation period is usually two days but it may be as short as one day or as long as seven. In about two-thirds of cases the onset is sudden, the first symptoms being a headache, a general feeling of illness, and either chilliness or feverishness. Within a few hours the body temperature rises to about 39 °C (101 °F) and often goes higher. A short, dry cough is one of the most regular signs. Those symptoms ordinarily associated with a common cold, such as sneezing, nasal blocking and discharge, and sore throat are only present in about 50 per cent of cases of influenza and are seldom prominent. Aching of the muscles of the back and legs

11

is an important feature of many cases and there may be pains in the joints. The eyes are often painful and watery. Occasionally there is nausea and vomiting but diarrhoea is rare.

In the classical disease the fever lasts three days but this may vary from one to six days. Sometimes after the temperature has subsided there is a secondary but lower elevation, resulting in the so-called diphasic fever-curve. This diphasic curve is also seen in ferrets which have been inoculated with the virus.

Although the acute phase of the illness is normally over after three to five days, there frequently remains a cough, lassitude, and a depressed feeling for one or two weeks longer. If the temperature remains high after the fourth or fifth day it probably means there are pulmonary complications.

The illness due to influenza virus type A is indistinguishable from that due to the type B virus except that the latter is often milder. The main features which distinguish influenza clinically from the common cold are fever, aches and pains, and a general feeling of illness and depression.

The clinical picture of the typical case is broadly similar in all epidemics but there may be some variation. Sometimes there is a greater tendency to develop pneumonia, more severe mental depression during convalescence or more frequent nausea and vomiting.

Influenza is primarily a respiratory disease, that is to say, in most cases the virus infects only the cells lining the nose, throat, trachea, and lungs. It has been generally thought that the muscular and joint pains are caused by the absorption of the products of cellular damage in the respiratory tract rather than by spread of the virus throughout the body. However, there is now some doubt whether this view is correct. In exceptional cases the virus can be found in blood, heart muscle, and brain.

The people who do not become ill during a pandemic or epidemic do not necessarily escape infection. Many people become infected without becoming ill or they are only slightly indisposed. The number of subclinical infections (those that are extremely mild or quite symptomless) is commonly about the same as the number of clinical cases, but the ratio varies in different outbreaks by as much as 4:1 to 1:7. These infections help influenza spread and they produce immunity in those fortunate enough to cope with the virus in this way. The innocuous nature of these infections can be shown in some instances to be due to the person having been partly immune, and in others it is thought to be due to the person having received only a very small dose of virus, but there is still much that we do not know about this subject.

If there are no complications the most important treatment is rest in bed. Aspirin is often prescribed to alleviate the symptoms but there is no evidence at all that it affects the course of the disease. Antibiotics and sulpha drugs should be used against complications due to bacterial infection but they have no effect whatever on the virus.

Much research effort has been devoted to developing drugs that act on the virus but there has been only limited success so far. It is now some years since a synthetic antiviral drug called amantadine was first introduced. It has been shown to have beneficial effects in animals, and controlled trials with naturally-occurring cases of influenza in man showed that amantadine hastened recovery but not dramatically so. This drug has not come into general use because it causes some undesirable side effects, though these are said not to be serious. Promising results have been obtained with some new antiviral drugs that are not yet on the market. The time may not be far off when effective drugs are available for the treatment of influenza.

The cardinal rules for dealing with uncomplicated influenza remain (1) confinement to bed at least during the duration of the fever, and (2) rest during convalescence. If either of these rules is broken the risk of developing complications and prolonging the ill effects of the disease is much increased. The importance of rest is confirmed by experience of influenza in horses which is exactly analogous to the human disease. If the horse is not rested until it is completely recovered the likelihood of it developing bronchitis and pneumonia is much greater.

GRIEVOUS EFFECTS

In a small proportion of cases, which varies according to the age group and to the outbreak, pneumonia develops. Occasionally it comes on suddenly in the early stage of the disease but more commonly it develops later due to a secondary bacterial infection. The frequency of pneumonia starts rising from the age of 50 and it rises steeply in the older age groups. Most influenzal deaths are due to pneumonia; the introduction of antibiotics and sulpha drugs has considerably reduced this mortality.

People with chronic bronchitis are particularly vulnerable to influenza, as are also those with chronic heart or kidney complaints. It is often severe in pregnant women and there is an increased risk of pneumonia and death compared to non-pregnant women. In most pandemics up to and including that of 1918–19, there were reports of abortions and stillbirths due to influenza. In 1918–19, one series of 1350 pregnant women who had influenza were observed: abortion, stillbirth or premature labour occurred in 26 per cent of those without pneumonia and 52 per cent of those with pneumonia. The prognosis was said to be serious for the women who aborted or went into labour. However, during the 1957–58 and 1968–69 pandemics and the epidemics in between, hardly any increase in abortions or stillbirths was reported.

It is of interest to note that in the 1918–19 pandemic the illness in the great majority of cases presented the characteristic picture of influenza. Even in the severe autumn wave 80 per cent of patients suffered only the usual 3–5 day illness. However, often the sudden onset was more striking than usual and I can remember some boys at my school collapsing suddenly and having to be carried to bed. It was commonly found that about 20 per cent of cases developed pneumonia and a considerable proportion of these – up to half – ended fatally. Frequently the pneumonia came on suddenly and some patients quickly developed a heliotrope colouration of the lips and face. Most of these patients did not feel especially ill and many remained cheerful but the doctors soon learnt that the heliotrope cyanosis nearly always meant death within 24 to 48 hours. This type of pneumonia, due to massive invasion of the lungs by the virus, has been seen occasionally during more recent epidemics.

A serious, but fortunately fairly rare, late effect of influenza B has only recently been recognized. In 1963, R. D. K. Reye of Sydney, Australia, described 21 cases of a disease affecting young children and characterized by acute degenerative changes in the brain, liver, and kidneys. Since then this syndrome has been diagnosed elsewhere and in 1973–74, in the U.S.A., 286 cases were reported of which 36 per cent died. There is good evidence that most, if not all, cases of Reye's syndrome, as it is now called, are caused by influenza B. The majority of cases have been found to have had that infection a week or ten days earlier.

Another possibly sinister aspect of influenza is that it might cause congenital defects, though this has not yet been definitely proved. There have been reports that defects, particularly of the brain, have followed infection with influenza during early pregnancy. Surveys have been carried out after epidemics of influenza but the results have been inconsistent. Some interesting research that has a bearing on this matter has been carried out on guinea-pigs. When their body temperature was raised experimentally during early pregnancy, some aborted and others produced offspring with various deformities. After the body temperature had been raised by 2.5 °C (4.5 °F) or by 3.3 °C (5.9 °F) some of the progeny appeared physically normal except that their brains were smaller than average. When animals affected in this way became adults and were subjected to psychological tests, it was found that their learning ability was below normal.

It seems probable that hyperthermia during early pregnancy has untoward effects in all species including man, and preliminary experiments in monkeys give some support to that view. This research has worrying implications for any febrile illness in pregnant women and influenza is one of the commonest single causes of fever in developed countries today. When one also recalls that influenza may be of more than average severity in pregnant women and that there may possibly be an increased risk of abortion, it seems to me that women who are pregnant or expecting to become so should be vaccinated, but with a killed vaccine. However, at present this is not the official recommendation in most countries; I suggest the authorities concerned should reconsider the recommendations.

PANDEMICS, EPIDEMICS, LOCAL OUTBREAKS, AND SPORADIC CASES

The most striking feature of the epidemic behaviour of influenza is that periodically pandemics occur that affect a large part of the world's population. The word pandemic means simply a widespread epidemic, but in the case of influenza, virologists now restrict the term to mean a world-wide epidemic caused by a new subtype of influenza virus type A. The most recent pandemics have been the Asiatic (1889–90), the Spanish (1918–19), the Asian (1957–58), and the Hong Kong (1968–69), which are described in the next chapter.

During the intervals between pandemics there are usually epidemics every one, two or three years. Some of these epidemics are limited to certain regions but some are world-wide. These latter could be described as pandemics according to the dictionary definition of the word, but since the virus involved is not a new subtype they do not qualify as influenza pandemics, so I shall refer to them as 'ordinary' epidemics, for want of a better term. The virus causing them is usually a new variant of the subtype that caused the preceding pandemic. Generally these epidemics do not affect such a high percentage of the population as pandemics, but there have been exceptions.

Influenza epidemics, both pandemics and severe 'ordinary' epidemics, have special characteristics that enable us to recognize them from historical descriptions. They often start suddenly and spread through the whole country in a month or so; they spread throughout continents and usually the whole world; people of all ages and walks of life are affected; many become ill but relatively few die and those are mainly the old or chronically sick; the illness frequently has a sudden onset and it takes the form of a fever commonly lasting about three days and accompanied by a cough and aches in the head, back, and legs; after the fever there may be weakness and depression for a week or more. The attack rate and the death rate vary from one epidemic to another, as well as between different countries and age groups, but broadly speaking the picture is similar – a very high attack rate, especially in pandemics, and a relatively low case fatality with the overall result of quite a large number of deaths.

Influenza has behaved in much the same way for hundreds of years except that in Britain there was a period of some forty years before the 1889–90 pandemic when influenza was at a low ebb, although there were epidemics elsewhere. Since 1889 there are good records showing that only on rare occasions have influenza epidemics been absent for more than two years. During the period from 1934 to 1968 there was a fairly regular pattern of influenza type A epidemics occurring at intervals of two or three years. Since the Hong Kong subtype of virus arrived in 1968 it has caused epidemics practically every year in most countries. In addition influenza virus type B epidemics have occurred at cycles of three to six years. Type A and type B cycle quite independently of each other and occasionally their epidemics have occurred at the same time.

When a new subtype of influenza virus type A arrives, the previous subtype disappears, as will be explained in Chapter 6. Therefore the 'ordinary' epi-

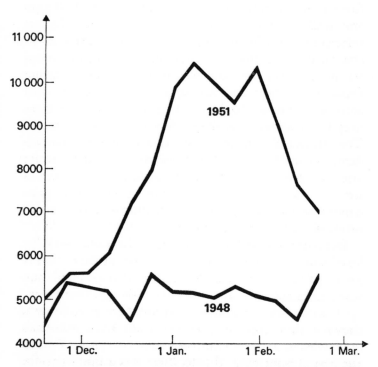

An example of the effect of influenza on the overall mortality. In the winter of 1950–51 there was an 'ordinary' epidemic, in 1947–48 there was not. In December, January, and February 1947–48 in 126 large towns in England and Wales there were between 4500 and 5700 deaths a week which may be regarded as normal, whereas in 1950–51 the figures were between 9000 and 10 500 for six weeks. (Data from W. H. Bradley, Proc. roy. Soc. Med., 1951, 44, 789.)

demics following each pandemic are all due to the same subtype as the preceding pandemic. Thus since 1957 the pandemic and its subsequent followers until 1968 were due to the Asian virus and its variants, and since 1968 the Hong Kong virus and its variants have been responsible for the pandemic and the subsequent recrudescences (except of course for the independent epidemics of influenza type B which are less frequent and less severe).

Influenza sometimes occurs as a local outbreak. These episodes happen mainly in closed or semi-closed communities such as orphanages, boarding schools, summer holiday camps, army training camps or prisons. Local outbreaks are seen when the strain of virus is not an aggressive spreader or the circumstances are not sufficiently favourable for an epidemic to occur. Apparently airborne spread is facilitated in compact communities and, in the case of schools, the children are more susceptible than the general population. Christopher Andrewes has suggested that institutional outbreaks may sometimes be due to a few of the people first infected being what he calls 'super-shedders'. Influenza type B is commonly limited to this type of outbreak, but institutional outbreaks with type A may be the prelude to a general epidemic.

Even in the absence of an outbreak a few sporadic cases of influenza can be detected at most times if one undertakes a laboratory investigation of a large number of cases of respiratory illness. Most 'off season' sporadic cases of influenza are in children. Nevertheless severe cases of the common cold are only exceptionally due to the influenza virus even though they may be diagnosed as such by a physician.

WAVES DURING PANDEMICS

It has often been said that it is a common characteristic of influenza pandemics that they occur in several waves. This was certainly true of the 1918–19 pandemic, which was exceptional in so many respects, but scrutiny of the other three pandemics of the last 100 years shows that this concept may be misleading.

After the onset of the 1889–90 pandemic, the so-called waves had their peaks in January 1890, March 1891, January 1892, and December 1893, that is, each occurred in a different winter. It is partly a question of semantics, but nowadays we would usually refer to such episodes as separate epidemics.

In 1918–19 there was a mild wave in the spring, an extremely severe one in the autumn, and a severe one early in 1919. All three were over within a period of twelve months in any one country. We do not know whether or not these waves were caused by the same virus subtype. In some communities people affected in the first or second wave turned out to be immune to attack in the subsequent wave(s), but in other communities this was not so. Possibly there were two different subtypes involved or else widely different variants of the same subtype.

It has been said that in the 1957–58 pandemic in the U.S.A., there were two waves because there was a peak of mortality in October 1957 and a smaller secondary peak the following February. However, the latter peak was not accompanied by the other accepted characteristics of epidemic influenza such as school and industrial absenteeism. Apparently what happened was that in the autumn the disease affected mainly the younger age groups; the virus continued to circulate and took its toll

in older adults and elderly people three to four months
later, possibly due to the colder weather.

The Hong Kong subtype caused major epidemics in
the winters of 1968 and 1969 and to a lesser extent most
winters since then. Some writers refer to these episodes
as waves but it seems to me more in keeping with present
day terminology to regard outbreaks occurring in a
different winter as seperate epidemics.

THE COST

The cold facts given in this and the following chapter
convey little of the social and economic effects of a
severe influenza epidemic. We cannot attempt to
measure the cost of the disease in human misery or
estimate the tragedies of sudden bereavement. There
are no scales for weighing grief; I leave it to the
reader's imagination to interpret this aspect of the
statistics.

However, we can give some indication of the mone-
tary losses caused by even one of the less grave pandemics,
that of 1968–69. The first point to make is that the disruption of administration, industry, and services is much
more severe than the bare figures suggest, because there
are so many people absent through illness at the same
time. In other words the effect is more than what just
'the sum of the parts' would indicate. The Hong Kong
pandemic in the last three months of 1968 in the U.S.A.
is said to have cost $225M just in providing Medicare
for people 65 years and over suffering from influenza. To
this must be added the medical cost of those under 65
and, even more important, the losses due to the absence
from work of the millions of sick people. Roger Egeberg
of the U.S. Department of Health, Education, and

Welfare estimated that the total economic loss of that pandemic in the U.S.A. was $4600M. 1968

In view of these figures, the expenditure in 1976 of $100M by the U.S. Government on vaccine against 'swine' influenza seems a sensible precaution. After the outbreak at Fort Dix, New Jersey, nobody can deny that there is a possibility of a pandemic, even if the risk is not great, so the production of vaccine is a good insurance. Mass vaccination may prevent a pandemic starting and the whole world would benefit. Unfortunately some unforseen difficulties have arisen. In preliminary trials it was found that people under 20 years of age developed little antibody after being injected with vaccine that had been refined in the way that most influenza vaccines are nowadays. Less refined vaccines gave better immune response in young people but they produced unpleasant reactions in some children. At the time I am writing it seems that different vaccine will have to be provided for children.

A valuable consequence of the outbreak at Fort Dix has been that all concerned have had to face up to the practical problems of mass vaccination such as would be indicated to meet the next pandemic, which is sure to come sooner or later.

The economic aspects of influenza merit serious study.

3

The influenza chronicle

Studying the past helps us understand the present and prepare for likely future events. This applies particularly to influenza which has occurred periodically since ancient times. During the latter part of the last century there was a wave of interest in the history of influenza and four books* were published from which I have derived much of the information in this chapter. One of the authors, Ditmar Finkler, wrote that the behaviour of influenza 'borders on the miraculous and fills us with wonder and astonishment'; some of the mystery has gone but it is still a fascinating subject with many unknowns.

The disease masqueraded under various names before the present name was generally accepted. The Italians introduced the term influenza during an outbreak in 1504 when the disease was attributed to the influence (= 'influenza') of the stars. However, some later writers refer to 'influenza di freddo', influence of the cold. The

---

* Charles Creighton, *A History of Epidemics in Britain*, (London: Cambridge University Press, 1894).

Ditmar Finkler, *Influenza* in *Twentieth Century Practice*, Ed. T. L. Stedman, Vol. XV, (London: Sampson Low, Marston & Co., 1898).

August Hirsch, *Handbook of Geographical and Historical Pathology*, Vol. I, 1881. Translated by Charles Creighton, (London: New Sydenham Society, 1883).

E. Symes Thompson, *Influenza*, (London: Percival & Co., 1890).

24

name influenza was adopted by the English during the epidemic of 1742–43; nowadays the abbreviation 'flu' is commonly used. It was also during the eighteenth century that the French began calling the disease grippe. Here again there are two possible etymologies. Some say it arose during an epidemic that coincided with a plague of insects of that name but a more appropriate origin is given in French dictionaries, namely that it comes from the word 'gripper' to grip.

Influenza epidemics have distinctive characteristics that enable us to make retrospective diagnoses with reasonable assurance from historical accounts. Here is a description of an outbreak 400 years ago that could only be influenza. Lord Randolph wrote from Edinburgh to Lord Cecil at the end of November 1562:

'Maye it please your Honor, immediately upon the Quene's [Mary's] arivall here, she fell acquainted with a new disease that is common in this towne, called here the newe acquayntance, which passed also throughe her whole courte, neither sparinge lordes, ladies nor damoysells not so much as ether Frenche or English. It ys a plague in their heades that have yt, and a sorenes in their stomackes, with a great coughe, that remayneth with some longer, with others shorter tyme, as yt findeth apte bodies for the nature of the disease. The queen kept her bed six days. There was no appearance of danger, nor manie that die of the disease, excepte some olde folkes. My lord of Murraye is now presently in it, the lord of Lidlington hathe had it, and I am ashamed to say that I have byne free of it, seinge it seketh acquayntance at all men's handes.'

Some epidemics recorded as far back as the classical era can be identified as probably influenza, one of the first being reported in 412 B.C. by Hippocrates and by Livy. Quite a number of epidemics that were beyond reasonable doubt influenza were described in the middle ages and one that was probably a true pandemic took place in 1510. It is said to have come from Africa and spread throughout Europe. There were few deaths but the attack rate was high – the disease 'attacked at once and raged all over Europe not missing a family and scarce a person'. In 1580 a definite pandemic occurred, which was possibly the first global dissemination of the disease. It started in Asia and spread to Africa, Europe, and America. It was said to be of such fierceness 'that in the space of six weeks it afflicted almost all the nations of Europe, of whom hardly the twentieth person was free of the disease, and anyone who was so became an object of wonder to others in the place . . . Its sudden ending after a month, as if it had been prohibited was as marvellous as its sudden onset'. In Britain there were two waves, one in the summer and one in the autumn. In some cities the mortality was high, 9000 died in Rome and some Spanish cities were said to be 'nearly entirely depopulated by the disease'. It was customary at the time to treat patients with fever by bleeding them and this practice undoubtedly added greatly to the mortality, as was realized afterwards.

One of the distinguishing features of influenza is that it affects all types of people; this was reported on in 1693 when 'all conditions of persons were attacked . . . those who were very strong and hardy were taken in the same manner as the weak and spoiled . . . the youngest as well as the oldest'.

PANDEMICS 1700 TO 1900

The historical record brings home to us forcefully that pandemics have occurred at intervals since ancient times. It might give us some guidance to the future if we knew how frequently they occurred in past centuries. The records before the eighteenth century are too irregular to enable one even to attempt to draw up a complete chronicle of pandemics, but from then on in at least some countries they become increasingly systematic and detailed. I have examined critically the records since 1700 and attempted to interpret them in the light of present knowledge and in particular identify pandemics as we now conceive them in virological terms as distinct from 'ordinary' epidemics. This has involved a good deal of arbitrary judgement for the period up to 1889. In interpreting the historical records one has to bear in mind that absence of reports in many countries could be because there were no reporters rather than no disease. Also as one goes back in history not only was the population smaller but human travel was much less in volume and slower, so that dissemination of the virus from one continent to another could not occur on the scale and speed that it does in modern times; hence one must expect epidemics to behave differently in different centuries.

During the 200 years up to 1900 there were sixteen major epidemics that I have evaluated as best I can on the evidence available as either pandemics (✸) or possibly pandemics (✳). The following is a brief description of them with my grading. It must be emphasized that there were also many other epidemics which I have judged as definitely not pandemics.

✳ 1729-30
Influenza was widespread in Europe with a high attack rate and appreciable mortality. In London, where it was regarded as a new disease, the overall death rate was doubled; it was said that barely one per cent escaped the disease, and during September a thousand died from it each week.

✳ 1732–33

Influenza was world-wide. In Plymouth, England, it was
reported that some were seized suddenly, 'they fell down in
multitudes, scarce anyone escaped it.' In London the overall
mortality was trebled at the height of the outbreak. This was
a severe and very widespread epidemic. One report states
clearly that it started in Connecticut, U.S.A., in October but
there is also a report that it started in Moscow in November.

✳ 1742–43

Influenza was widespread in Europe. In Rome 80 000 people
were ill and as many as 500 people were buried there in one
day. In London the overall death rate was trebled at the
beginning of April.

✳ 1761–62

North America and the West Indies were affected in 1761
and Europe the following year. The mortality was variable;
it was high in Breslau in February 1762.

✳ 1767

Influenza was reported in all North America and most of
Europe but it was quite unimportant in Britain.

✳ 1775–76

All Europe and the Near and Far East were affected but there
was little mortality in England.

✳ 1781–82

Influenza was reported from all European countries, China,
India, and North America. Finkler wrote that this was one
of the most widespread pandemics of the disease that has ever
occurred. In St Petersburg [Leningrad], 30 000 fell ill each
day, in Rome two-thirds of the population were attacked, and
in Munich three-quarters. In London it caused an increase in
the death rate in June and it raged in other parts of Britain in
July and August. This unusual seasonal incidence is strong
evidence that it was a true pandemic quite apart from the fact
that it had a world-wide distribution. All reports state that it
started in China in the autumn.

✳ **1788–89**
Influenza occurred in North America and throughout Europe.
In Britain the illness was mild and caused hardly any deaths
and it was regarded as a recurrence of the 1781–82 disease.

✳ **1800–02**
All Europe, China, and Brazil were affected but the disease
was generally mild and little mortality resulted. It is difficult
to decide when and where this outbreak started as there
seems to have been influenza somewhere almost continuously
from 1800 to 1803; two historians say Russia in October and
one says China in September.

✳ **1830–33**
There was a general diffusion of the disease over the whole
world in the course of three years. In Britain it started in the
early summer of 1831 and there was a 'really serious influenza'
early in 1833. In London the overall death rate was nearly
quadrupled during the worst two weeks. All writers agree this
pandemic started in China in January.

✳ **1836–37**
Influenza occurred in Europe, parts of Africa, and in
Australia. There was considerable mortality in London. This
episode was probably a recurrence of the undoubted pandemic
of 1830–33.

✳ **1847–48**
Influenza was widespread in Europe, North America, the
West Indies, and Brazil. In Paris between a quarter and a half
of the people developed influenza. In Britain it was referred to
as 'the great influenza of 1847'; there was considerable
mortality and there were said to be 250 000 cases in London.
The ravages of the disease were compared to those from
cholera, as there were more influenza deaths than there had
been cholera deaths during the great epidemic of that disease
in 1832. It is not entirely clear where or when this pandemic
started but two historians say it started in March in
Russia.

✳ 1850–51
There was influenza in North and South America, the West Indies, Australia, and Germany. This was probably a recurrence or late extension of the 1847 pandemic.

✳ 1857–58
Influenza was widespread in North and South America and in Europe. Seifert referred to it as 'one of the greatest epidemics'. There were many deaths in Rome. However, in Britain the only report was 'a slight epidemic in Scotland' which casts some doubt on its classification as a true pandemic. All writers say it started in Panama in August.

✳ 1873–75
Influenza was widespread in North America and the European Continent but again Britain was not affected.

✳ 1889–90
This was the so-called Asiatic influenza pandemic. The first report was from Bukhara in Russia in May. At the start it spread very slowly and it was not till October that it reached Tomsk and the Caucasus. Then it spread rapidly westward and throughout the world. North America was invaded in December and South American countries between February and April. The eastern Mediterranean countries suffered in January, India in February and March, and Australia in March and April. There was a high attack rate everywhere with considerable mortality. In several German cities the incidence was said to be 40–50 per cent and from 0.5 to 1.2 per cent of the population died. In subsequent winters for several years there were severe epidemics due presumably to the same or a related virus.

THE GREAT PANDEMIC OF 1918–19

In all the history of influenza there is one event that stands out above all others – the great pandemic of so-called Spanish influenza of 1918–19. The possible origin of this pandemic is discussed in the next chapter.

There were three waves in less than twelve months. The first wave in the spring of 1918 was regarded as mild and the mortality was not unusually high. The attack rate varied with age as follows: 0–35 years, 30–40 per cent; 50 year olds, 20 per cent; 70 year olds, 10 per cent. As usual with influenza, most of the mortality was in old people, but there were also an appreciable number of deaths in the 20–40 age group. The second wave came in the autumn of 1918 and it was the most spectacular outbreak of any disease for hundreds of years. A unique and extraordinary feature was that about half the deaths were in the 20–40 year age group and this was the pattern throughout the world. The third wave early in 1919 was rather less severe but the age distribution of the deaths was similar.

The total mortality caused by the three waves in the U.S.A. was 0.5 per cent of the population – over 500 000 deaths. In England and Wales the official figure was 200 000 deaths and in most developed countries the mortality was of the same order. In a few places the mortality was much higher. In Samoa 25 per cent of the people died. The Eskimoes in Alaska suffered terribly; some villages were wiped out and others lost their entire adult population. In Nome 176 out of 300 Eskimoes died. The disease caused havoc in India where an estimated five million people died. In the Punjab the streets were littered with the dead and at railway stations the trains had to be cleared of dead and dying passengers. The burial grounds were covered with corpses.

In this pandemic, as in other influenza pandemics, people of all socioeconomic classes from kings to beggars suffered to much the same extent. However, the incidence sometimes varied considerably in different

communities. This was very noticeable among people
on ships at sea, for example on passenger liners arriving
in Australia during the pandemic the incidence varied
from 4 per cent to 43 per cent and the case fatality from
nil to 7 per cent. There were also great differences on
ships of the British Navy. In three English public schools
the attack rate varied from 22 to 67 per cent during the
autumn wave. The total deaths throughout the world
were estimated at between 15–25 million – the greatest
visitation ever experienced by the human race.

Warren Vaughan of the Harvard Medical School,
writing in the American Journal of Epidemiology of
1921, compared the mortality from influenza in the
American Army with that from other great plagues:

> 'This fatality has been unparallelled in recent times. The
> influenza epidemic of 1918 ranks well up with the epidemics
> famous in history. Epidemiologists have regarded the dis-
> semination of cholera from the Broad Street well in London
> as a catastrophe. The typhoid epidemic of Plymouth, Pa., of
> 1885, is another illustration of the damage that can be done
> by epidemic disease once let loose. Yet the fatality from
> influenza and pneumonia at Camp Sherman was greater than
> either of these. Compared with epidemics for which we have
> fairly accurate statistics the death rate at Camp Sherman in
> the fall of 1918 is surpassed only by that of plague in London
> in 1665 and that of yellow fever in Philadelphia in 1793. The
> plague killed 14 per cent of London's population in seven
> months' time. Yellow fever destroyed 10 per cent of the
> population of Philadelphia in four months. In seven weeks
> influenza and pneumonia killed 3.1 per cent of the strength
> at Camp Sherman. If we consider the time factor, these three
> instances are not unlike in their lethality. The plague killed
> 2 per cent of the population in a month, yellow fever 2.5 per
> cent, and influenza and pneumonia 1.9 per cent.'

The 1918–19 pandemic was by far the most serious in
recent times and we have come to think of it as quite

exceptional. However, perhaps it is not unique. Judging from historical accounts, some epidemics in former times that may have been influenza were just as devastating.

PANDEMICS DURING THE VIROLOGICAL ERA

In 1946 a variant that differed markedly from previous strains was detected in Australia; it became world-wide but did not give rise to a major epidemic. Kilbourne and others classified this episode as a pandemic but this does not seem justified in the light of antigenic analysis of influenza viruses during the last few years, which indicates that the 1946 virus was not a new subtype, nor from the character of the epidemic.

In 1957 the pandemic of Asian influenza arose in China. It started in western Kweichow and eastern Yunnan in February and reached Europe and the U.S.A. in June. In the U.S.A. the attack rate the following winter in several surveys was from 50 to 70 per cent for the 10 to 20 years age group, 20 to 40 per cent between the ages of 20 and 50 years, and it was lower again in older people. Although this incidence of the disease was higher than in any epidemic for some years, the mortality was no greater. Some 60 000 deaths were attributed to Asian influenza over the six month period October 1957 to March 1958 in the U.S.A. A majority of the deaths were in people over 65 years of age. The statistics for mortality were about the same in most countries but were somewhat higher in Japan and considerably higher in Finland.

In 1968 the pandemic caused by the Hong Kong virus started in south-east China in July. During the following winter in the U.S.A. all age groups were attacked to about the same extent – 30–40 per cent according to one survey but only 15 per cent according to another. The mortality in the U.S.A. was estimated at around 80 000. The disease behaved very differently in Europe. There the attack rate was about the same as in the U.S.A. but, surprisingly, hardly any mortality could be attributed to influenza that winter. However, when the disease recurred the next winter (1969–70) there was considerable mortality in Europe with an estimated 30 000 deaths in an 8 week period in Britain alone. During the week ending 2 January 1970 there were 3170 influenza deaths in England and Wales distributed between the age groups as follows: 0–44 years, 144 deaths; 45–64 years, 753 deaths; 65–74 years, 1362 deaths; 75 and over, 911 deaths. In the U.S.A. the mortality was less in the winter of 1969–70.

During the interval between pandemics there have been many epidemics which, though commonly less widespread or dramatic, have often caused much illness and mortality, sometimes even more than the pandemics themselves. In England during the 1932–33 epidemic influenzal deaths rose to 2000 a week and during the 1967–68 epidemic, before the Hong Kong virus arrived, 18 000 deaths were attributed to influenza during an 8 week period.

Occasionally the second outbreak of a subtype has caused more deaths than the first. As mentioned above, this was so with the Hong Kong virus in Europe in 1968–70. During the 1918 pandemic the second wave was much more severe than the first but in this case we are not sure that the same subtype was involved in both waves. During the pandemic of Asiatic influenza in 1889–90 there was a high incidence of illness but not many deaths during the first outbreak, but when the

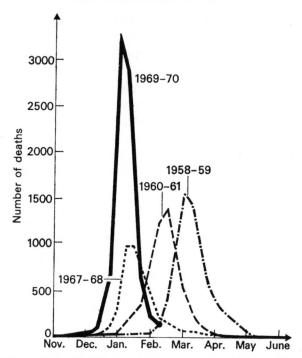

Influenza deaths in England and Wales. The epidemic in 1969–70 was due to the Hong Kong virus, the three previous epidemics were due to variants of the Asian virus, but influenza type B contributed to the deaths in 1958–59. (Brit. Med. Journal, 1970, 1, 507.)

disease, presumably due to the same subtype, recurred the two following winters there were many more deaths although fewer people fell ill. The reason for a second outbreak sometimes causing more deaths might be that the virus has developed greater virulence. Alternatively it is conceivable that following an attack one becomes sensitized to that subtype and subsequent invasion by a new but related variant of it sometimes leads to the immune mechanism over-reacting.

LOOKING FORWARD

As with all natural phenomenon that occur periodically, many people have attempted to discern a pattern of regular cycles with influenza on which to base predictions, but the data are as recalcitrant as are those on the weather (which incidentally may have a bearing on influenza).

The intervals between dates of onset of the twenty major epidemics described varied from 3 to 28 years, which gives an average of about 12 years. However, I consider it unlikely that many of the episodes graded only ✳ were truly pandemics. If we accept just those graded ✳ before 1900 and the unquestioned pandemics of this century, the intervals vary from 10 to 49 years, the average being about 24 years. The only conclusion we can reach is that pandemics have occurred at very irregular intervals averaging somewhere between 12 and 24 years.

Some virologists have predicted that we are likely to experience pandemics about every decade from now on. Two points are advanced in support of this view. First, the interval between the last two pandemics was eleven years (1957–68), and second, pandemics should occur at shorter intervals now than before the Second World War because the vast amount of travel that takes place will promote rapid dissemination of virus. It is argued that quicker exhaustion of susceptibles to the prevailing subtype will favour the emergence of a new subtype. This may be true but we still have a great deal to learn about influenza and experience has shown that predictions about it have seldom proved correct.

The one definite conclusion arising from studies of the long and diverse history of this capricious virus is

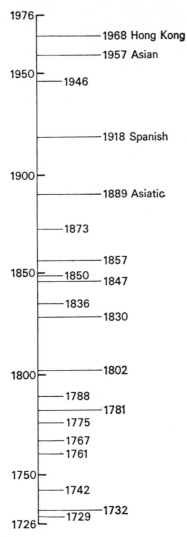

Pandemics during the last 250 years. The long lines represent ten definite pandemics, the shorter lines ten possible pandemics. Between the pandemics there were many 'ordinary' epidemics that are not shown.

I.—4

that epidemics on a global scale will continue to occur until we devise and implement more effective measures of combating the disease than we have now. Charles Cockburn, writing as head of the virus section of the World Health Organization in 1973, said: 'The influenza virus behaves just as it seems to have done 500 or 1000 years ago and we are no more capable of stopping epidemics or pandemics than our ancestors were'.

4

The spread of infection

In Chapter 7 I shall discuss theories on *how* new sub-types of virus that give rise to pandemics come into existence. In this chapter I shall set out what information we have about *where* the births take place, or rather where they have in the past. Then I shall mention various factors that affect their spread.

In 1928 the epidemiologist Clifford Gill published a book called *The Genesis of Epidemics**, a subject he had studied intensively. In it he stated 'all authorities are agreed that pandemics of influenza can almost in- variably be traced to "the silent spaces" of Asia, Siberia and Western China'. Another notable authority on the subject, Charles Creighton, wrote in his *A History of Epidemics in Britain* published in 1894:

> 'In the early winter of 1889 the newspapers began to publish long telegrams on the influenza in Moscow, St Petersburg, Berlin, Paris, Madrid, and other foreign capitals. This epidemic wave, like those immediately preceding it . . . in 1833, 1837, and 1847, and like one or more, but by no means all, of the earlier influenzas, had an obvious course from Asiatic and European Russia towards Western Europe . . . The Russian Army Medical Report favoured the view that

* Clifford A. Gill, *The Genesis of Epidemics*, (London: Ballière, Tindall and Cox, 1928).

the birthplace of this pandemic in the autumn of 1889 was an extensive region occupied by nomadic tribes in the northern part of the Kirghiz Steppe. There is evidence of its rapid progress westwards over Tobolsk to the borders of European Russia.'

On many occasions epidemics have been called Russian influenza not only by the English, Germans, French, and Italians but also by the Chinese. Ironically the Russians have sometimes called the same epidemics Chinese fevers.

I have scrutinized the records about the primary focus – the starting point – of the seven pandemics that are graded ✳ in the preceding chapter and the three pandemics this century and the information available is summarized in Table 1. Four (or possibly five) were first reported in China, three (or possibly five) in Russia, one (or possibly two) in the U.S.A., one in Panama, and possibly one in Africa.

Table 1

Countries where pandemics were first reported

Country	Date pandemic started
China	1781, 1830, 1957, 1968, (possibly mild wave 1918).
Russia	1800, 1847, 1889, (possibly 1732, possibly severe wave 1918).
U.S.A.	1732, (possibly mild wave 1918).
Panama	1857
Africa	(possibly severe wave 1918).

It could well be that pandemics reported first in Russia or China started in Gill's 'silent spaces' and were only reported after they had reached the more populous and developed regions. The reports are certainly consistent

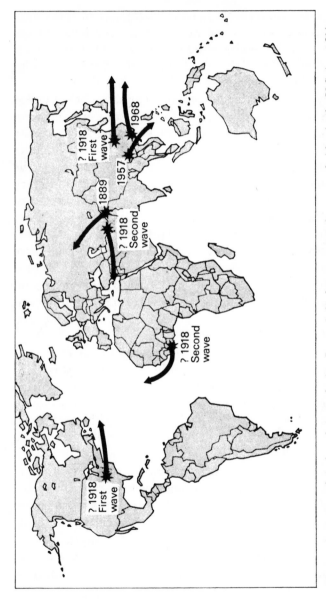

The starting points of the last four pandemics. In 1918 the first wave may have started either in the U.S.A. or China; the second, very severe wave, may have started in Russia or Sierra Leone.

with Gill's statement that the birthplace of most pandemics was somewhere not far from the heart of the great Eurasian landmass. The region implicated is vast. Some two or three thousand miles and enormous mountain ranges separate the eastern boundaries of European Russia from southern China. Surely there is some special significance in so many of the pandemics starting in this region; a possible explanation is offered in Chapter 7.

Let us look closer at the information concerning the origin of the important 1918–19 pandemic about which there is so much uncertainty. In the early spring of 1918 there were localized outbreaks of influenza in military camps in the U.S.A. and in April in France where the infection may have been carried by the American troops. The disease spread to Spain at the end of April where it received great publicity. It developed in England in June, where it was called Spanish influenza, and this misleading name stuck. This was the so-called 'mild spring wave'.

About the same time there were outbreaks on the other side of the world. Influenza was reported in March in China and in the Japanese Navy and by May it was widespread in China.

During 1918 there were brought together in Europe not only troops from all corners of the world but also large numbers of labourers from China and elsewhere. People were crowded together often under conditions of great misery, so circumstances were ideal for the exchange of infection and the start of an epidemic. (Circumstances were in many ways even worse in the Second World War but no pandemic arose then.)

In September the second wave swept Europe and within a few weeks virtually the whole population of the world was affected. This time the disease was much more severe and the mortality was high, especially in the 20–35 age group. The second wave lasted about six weeks in each city and then died down.

Attempts have also been made to ascertain the primary focus of the virulent second wave, as this may have been due to a quite different virus from that causing the mild spring wave. A severe outbreak with high mortality occurred in Meshed in Persia at the beginning of August; this was said to have come from Ashkhabad, a city in south-east Russia. At this time Russia was disorganized by revolution so we have no information on how influenza was behaving in that part of the world. Also in August, severe disease occurred on ships serving the west coast of Africa. An English ship, the H.M.S. *Africa*, left Sierra Leone for England and before it reached home 75 per cent of the ship's complement had become ill with influenza and 7 per cent had died; some other ships were similarly affected. In Bombay the severe form of the disease started in September.

It is impossible to reach any conclusion about the primary focus of the first wave in 1918 but the most likely places were the U.S.A. and China. The severe second wave may have evolved from the first – already an excessive number of deaths were occurring in young adults in June – or it may have been an invasion of a new virus from Russia or Africa.

It should be remembered that this discussion is concerned with the birthplace only of pandemics and takes no account of the many epidemics of lesser importance that occur at intervals of one, two or three years between pandemics. Between pandemics the virus is endemic, that is there is a trickle of infection passing around all the time and whenever the virus' characteristics have changed sufficiently and/or the general level of immunity of the population has fallen sufficiently, an epidemic springs up. This process can and does occur anywhere in the world and the actual starting point has not the special significance that attaches to the birthplace of a new pandemic subtype.

EFFECT OF SEASON

The history of the disease during previous centuries shows that the seasonal incidence of influenza has always been much the same as it has been during the twentieth century, that is, epidemics are much more common during the cold months of the years but occasionally they occur in the summer. The peak of epidemics in the northern hemisphere is usually January or February, though they not infrequently start in November or December, and in the southern hemisphere the main influenza season is June, July, and August. Most summer outbreaks have been due to the introduction of a new pandemic strain. Tropical countries are not spared during epidemics.

It is not completely known why influenza has this predilection for winter but there are several factors which are believed to play a part. Probably the most important one is that in cold weather people spend more time indoors, there are more indoor crowds, and the buildings are less well ventilated. These circumstances facilitate aerial transmission of the virus. The spread of influenza is greatly influenced by the density and mass of a population; it spreads exceptionally well in concentrated communities such as institutionalized groups – orphanages, training camps, the crews of naval ships. Another factor aiding spread in winter is that there is more sneezing and coughing in cold weather, partly because low temperature itself often has this effect and partly because common colds are more prevalent then. A third factor may be the longer hours of sunshine and higher temperature in the summer which militate against the survival of the virus in the air.

Some interesting experiments have been carried out on mice. While J. L. Schulman and E. D. Kilbourne of New York were experimenting with the spread of influenza in groups of mice, they found that the season the work was carried out greatly affected the results. Between July and October only one out of 120 contact mice became infected whereas in December and January forty-eight out of 216 contracted the disease. After that they did their experiments under conditions where the temperature and humidity were strictly controlled. With a temperature of 22 °C (72 °F) and a relative humidity of 50 per cent transmission was successful all the year round, but still there was some seasonal difference, 34 per cent of takes in the summer compared to 58 per cent in the winter. They did not identify the remaining factor operating.

Whether or not people are in themselves more susceptible in the winter than the summer is a moot point on which there has been much discussion but at present there is no unequivocal evidence that they are. Many writers still use the non-commital term 'winter factor' so as to leave open the possibility that some as yet unidentified factor plays a part in making influenza more prevalent in winter.

It is interesting to note that influenza in horses does not follow the same seasonal trends as in man. Most outbreaks have been in the spring and autumn. A likely explanation is that there are fewer sporting events in the winter and therefore less opportunity for the infection to spread from one riding school or training establishment to another. Generally the horses kept at one stable have no contact with horses at other stables except when taking part in sporting events. Considering the relatively sparse population of horses today and the fact that almost the only opportunities for transmission of infection from one group to another are open-air gatherings without crowding, it is remarkable that equine influenza can still flourish as it does.

The information available about the time of year that the pandemics described in Chapter 3 started is summarized in Table 2. In view of the fact that influenza occurs most often in the winter, it is surprising that only two of the eleven first reports refer to winter months whereas three refer to spring, three to summer, and three to autumn. Even allowing that some of these reports may not accurately reflect the commencement of a pandemic, the data seems at least to justify the conclusion that pandemics have most often started outside the winter months. It is difficult to guess what significance lies behind the apparent fact that pandemics do not usually start in the season of greatest prevalence.

Table 2

Seasons when pandemics were first reported

Winter:	January 1830, February 1957
Spring:	March 1847, May 1889, March 1918 (mild wave)
Summer:	August 1857, August 1918 (severe wave), July 1968
Autumn:	October/November 1732, 'Autumn' 1781, September/October 1800

Nevertheless this is useful information to have when one is conducting surveillance of influenza.

SPREAD THROUGH THE AIR

Although it is now generally believed that an epidemic, however alarming its spread may be, does not travel faster than can be explained by person to person contagion, there have been sudden mass outbreaks where this explanation did not appear adequate to contemporary observers. Also there have been reports of influenza attacking the crews of ships at sea without contact with ports where the disease was evident. One of the most striking of these puzzling episodes concerned an English warship *Arachne* in 1857. She was cruising off the coast of Cuba 'without any contact with land'. No less than 114 men out of a crew of 149 fell ill with influenza and only later was it learnt that there had been outbreaks in Cuba at the same time. The official report included the remark: 'A question therefore arises whether it might not have been caused by infection wafted from the shore.'

Before we discuss reports of this nature any further, it may help the reader if I outline modern concepts of airborne infection. When one sneezes or coughs thousands of droplets are blown into the air and some will be inhaled by anybody who is nearby. However, most of the droplets quickly dry out to become 'droplet nuclei' which can float about in the air for hours. Droplet nuclei are minute particles of dried mucus or saliva and they contain any viruses or bacteria that may be present in the respiratory tract and mouth of the person emitting them. The influenza virus is able to live for many hours in droplet nuclei provided they are not exposed to sunlight. When inhaled some droplet nuclei are retained in the nose and some pass right down into the lungs. This is the way influenza passes from one person to another.

Inside a building droplet nuclei are carried around by air currents and it is quite possible for someone to pick up infection from another person in a different room. Also trains, buses, underground stations, cinemas, and indeed any enclosed space facilitate the aerial spread of virus.

In the open air the infection becomes diluted and may be exposed to sunlight which is lethal to it. Therefore the likelihood of transmission is much less out of doors and it used to be thought virtually non-existent over distances more than a few feet. However, during recent years it has been found that two virus diseases of animals – Newcastle disease of chickens and foot-and-mouth disease of cloven hoofed animals – sometimes spread many kilometres from one farm to another on the wind.

In the light of these well-authenticated modern observations one cannot dismiss the possibility that influenza virus may be carried for some distance on the wind on cold nights, which is the time when conditions are favourable for virus survival. However, dissemination of the virus in this way, if it occurs at all, does so probably only exceptionally. Evidence against it happening commonly is provided by reports that during the 1890 pandemic people in 21 prisons in Germany and 39 in England remained free of influenza. Many of the outbreaks reported on ships at sea may have been due to people having been taken on board who were infected with influenza but did not show symptoms. Explosive mass outbreaks on land could be explained as following crowd gatherings in which there were some people shedding virus. It is quite understandable that a crowd in a building could be infected from just a few people. It could even happen at out-of-door gatherings as it certainly does with horses.

The rapidity of spread of influenza is related to its very short incubation period of only one to three days and the fact that the virus multiplies in the surface membranes of the respiratory tract from which it is readily shed into the air. Shedding of virus starts about 24 hours after exposure to infection. Shedding continues for only about a week, so the virus must either spread quickly or risk dying out.

SLOW-STARTING PANDEMICS

In view of the capacity of influenza to spread rapidly, one might expect that as soon as a new pandemic strain invades a country it would immediately run wild, as the population is fully susceptible. Sometimes this happens but often there is a delay of several months before the outbreak gets under way. We have to seek explanations for these different types of behaviour.

Many years ago Richard Shope was struck by the explosive nature of some outbreaks of influenza in people and in swine and he did not believe that the behaviour of the disease could be explained by the conventional view of case-to-case transmission. He raised the same objections as Charles Creighton and others did in the last century, but Shope offered a different explanation. He postulated that widespread 'pre-seeding' of virus occurred without causing disease. The virus was supposed to be in a 'masked' form in which it was innocuous. Later these latent infections were simultaneously activated by some stress factor such as the onset of cold weather, resulting in an explosive outbreak affecting many centres at the same time. Shope's ideas about masked viruses have not been generally accepted but the concept of pre-seeding some time in advance of a pandemic has been adopted by many epidemiologists. There is commonly a latent period of some months during which the pandemic seems to hang fire; small isolated outbreaks occur where people are concentrated into groups such as in schools, army training centres, summer camps or even congresses, but there is no spread in the general population.

Edwin Kilbourne, a leading influenza researcher and editor of an authoritative book on the disease published in 1975*, states that there is no doubt that pandemic influenza smoulders before it bursts into flame. He supports this statement by outlining events following the introduction of the Asian and the Hong Kong viruses into the U.S.A. in 1957 and 1968.

There seem to me two likely explanations for the slow development of pandemics: first, a change in the transmissibility of the virus, and second, and more important, the seasonal effect.

The new pandemic subtype may not at first have acquired the maximum degree of transmissibility in man. It could well be that the infectivity of the virus is enhanced as it passes through a series of people, by a process of mutation and selection, or even perhaps by hybridization with the old subtype. This enhancement happens when we transmit a virus repeatedly in a new host in the laboratory. Furthermore we know that

* Edwin D. Kilbourne, ed. *The Influenza Viruses and Influenza.* (New York: Academic Press, 1975).

pandemic strains do sometimes change in other respects during the course of a pandemic, such as gaining in virulence and developing slightly different immunological characteristics.

However, quite apart from possible changes in the virus, I think that the delay period in 1957 and in 1968 can simply be explained by the fact that the viruses arrived in America and Europe 'out of season', that is, at a time of the year unfavourable for widespread dissemination to occur. The facts are described below.

The origin of the 1957 Asian virus was traced retrospectively to south-west China where cases of the disease first appeared in early February. Possibly retarded by restricted travel, it took two months to reach Hong Kong where it caused an outbreak in April and was recognized as a new subtype. In May the virus spread to south-east Asia and Japan, and isolated cases were recognized in Europe and the U.S.A. in June. The most rapid spread was in the populations of the tropical countries of Asia. In Japan there was an epidemic from May until July which then died down but recurred in September and lasted until December. The Japanese experience could be regarded as two waves or as one epidemic temporarily interrupted by the arrival of the summer season. In the U.S.A. the first indigenous cases were diagnosed 2 June and the first outbreak started in a girls' camp in California on 20 June. During the following weeks there were fifteen camp outbreaks but it was not until September that the epidemic spread throughout the country.

In 1968 the first report of the new virus was in July in China and Hong Kong. In August it caused epidemics in Singapore and the Philippines. It was introduced in Japan a number of times but failed to spread

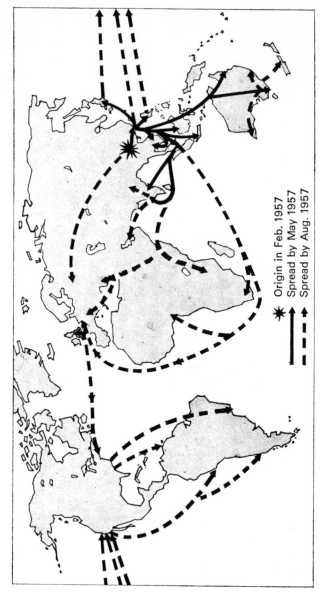

The spread of Asian influenza around the world. It started in China in February 1957 and reached Hong Kong in April. The solid black lines indicate the spread up until May, the broken lines the spread up until August. (Data from Chronicle of World Health Organization, Sept. 1957.)

Origin in Feb. 1957
Spread by May 1957
Spread by Aug. 1957

there until the winter. The virus was introduced to America and caused a localized outbreak in California in October; it spread widely in November and caused an epidemic that reached a peak about Christmas. In Europe the rise in incidence began later than in the U.S.A. and continued in some countries until the following April.

The circumstances seem to have been in many ways similar at the beginning of the 1889 pandemic in Russia. The first recognized outbreak was in Bukhara, Uzbekistan, in May and it is said to have been confined to that city until August. Then it slowly travelled to Siberia where it caused an outbreak at Tomsk in October. About the same time it appeared in the Caucasus and in European Russia. Later in October it reached Moscow and St Petersburg [Leningrad]. A month later it was in many European countries and in December it reached America. In January it was in Mexico, Egypt, Japan, and South Africa.

In all three of these pandemics the slow initial progress was connected with the warm season of the year, and the subsequent rapid dissemination with the arrival of the cooler months. Thus the seasonal effect provides an adequate explanation for the early behaviour of these pandemics but this does not exclude the possibility that some enhancement of the virus was also taking place during the latent period.

Clearly there is still much to learn about the epidemiology of influenza.

5

Influenza in animals

In the history of influenza it is extraordinary how many reports there are that horses were affected with apparently the same disease as the people during epidemics. Other species are also mentioned but less frequently. This is what August Hirsch wrote in his *Handbook of Geographical and Historical Pathology*, in 1881:

> 'I am not of the opinion that there is any question of accident in *the relation of influenza epidemics to epizootics of the same character prevailing at the same time*, especially among horses, and, next to them, among dogs, cats, and the like. Even in the oldest epidemiological records, there are indications of these coincidences both as regards time and place, as well as the identity or at least similarity of the form of disease; and the number of these observations is so remarkably large that the suggestion of an etiological connection between the epidemics on the one hand, and those epizootics on the other, may be regarded as provisionally proved.'
> (The italics are his.)

The English epidemiologist Clifford Gill wrote in 1928 that there is a traditional belief that horses are invariably affected during influenza epidemics. The association of respiratory disease in animals with influenza in man has been so striking that some epidemiologists, cited by Charles Creighton, have used it as evidence indicating that an epidemic that occurred

54

during the siege of Troy was influenza 'because it began upon the horses and dogs as so many historic influenzas have done'.

During the eighteenth and nineteenth centuries outbreaks of influenza-like illness in horses are reported to have been associated with human influenza epidemics in each of the following twelve epidemic years: 1728, 1733, 1737, 1750, 1760, 1767, 1771, 1775, 1788, 1837, 1857, and 1890. Until about the middle of the last century, however, ideas about the specificity and causes of infectious diseases were vague and it was a common practice to relate outbreaks of human disease to any event happening at the same time such as natural phenomena and diseases in animals. Many of these reports we now regard as mere coincidences and fanciful speculations. Clearly we must look with considerable scepticism on old records connecting human and animal influenza, nevertheless, as Hirsch remarked, the reports are so frequent and the disease in horses is so similar that I feel we cannot ignore these reports. The connection between human influenza and horse influenza seems too strong to be dismissed as only coincidence even if the less frequent accounts involving other species might mostly be regarded as such. The description of the clinical disease in horses and its epidemiology are usually typical of influenza. Of particular interest are the reports that the horses were often affected a month or so before the people, the implication being that the infection passed from horse to man possibly taking some weeks to become adapted. It is worth quoting some of these reports. In 1688 a doctor writing about the 'horse cold' then prevalent said that 'before the fever began [in the people] a slight but universal disease seized the horses'. In 1728 and 1733 'a most severe cough seized

almost all the horses one or two months before the men'.
In 1775 'catarrh' was prevalent in the horses in England,
'this "distemper" prevailed some time among horses
before it attacked the human species. The cough har-
assed them severely and rendered them unfit for work,
though few died.'

The pandemic of 1889–90 is of special interest in this
connection because there is some evidence from modern
'serological archaeology' (described in Chapter 6) indicating that the virus we now know as influenza
A/equine 2 may have affected people about the time of
that pandemic. In 1890, Symes Thompson wrote: 'So
strongly impressed were we with the intimate connection between "pink-eye" in horses and human influenza
that in the early part of December 1889 . . . the author
wrote to the British Medical Journal calling attention
to the prevalence of an epidemic among horses and
suggesting it would not improbably prove the fore-
runner of an outbreak in man. Subsequent events fully
justified this forecast'. The forecast was correct only
in so far as a human pandemic did start in London in
December, but there can be no doubt that it originated
from Russia and not from the outbreak in English
horses. There were, however, several instances where
the circumstances suggested that people and horses
shared the same infection. Judging from contemporary
accounts it seems likely that there were two diseases
affecting horses about that time, one of which may have
been influenza, but the whole situation is very confused.
Although the disease was not introduced to the people
in London from horses, there may have been some
exchange of infection between men and horses.

It must of course be borne in mind that the horse
population was very much greater before they were

largely replaced by the internal combustion engine after the First World War. Furthermore there were large numbers of horses in the cities in close contact with people.

Turning now to the present century, I have already described in Chapter 1 the recognition of influenza in swine in the Midwest of the U.S.A. Also in the autumn of 1918 a Hungarian veterinarian, Altmann Aladár, described a disease in pigs which he believed was influenza. His description agrees well with Koen's and was of course quite independent. The only report of influenza in horses during the 1918 pandemic was by three French veterinarians. They reported outbreaks of coughing in several villages at the same time as influenza affected the people and they recalled a severe epidemic in horses during the 1889 pandemic.

During the 1918–19 pandemic there were also reports of baboons dying in large numbers in South Africa, and of widespread mortality in bison, elk, and other big game in North America. There was an epidemic among sheep in the county of Westmorland, England, that was considered to be influenza by a veterinarian with thirty years experience of sheep diseases.

However, during the first half of this century scientists showed little interest in influenza of animals excepting for the swine influenza in the U.S.A. Following Shope's work there was one isolation of influenza from pigs at Cambridge, England, in 1941, but surveys carried out in 1948 and later indicated that the infection had died out in Britain. Generally the earlier reports of influenza in animals were discounted and influenza came to be regarded as an exclusively human disease, excepting only for the pigs which had caught it from man. Also it was pointed out that the pig is an animal that has much in common with man from a physiological point of view, so it was rather a special case.

THE BREAKTHROUGH

Unfortunately the term 'influenza' had become attached to a disease of horses that we now know as infectious arteritis or 'pink-eye' This disease bears only a superficial resemblance to human influenza, so veterinarians dismissed the idea that there was any connection between influenza in people and in horses. It was well known that horses were also subject to epizootics of a respiratory disease which was referred to as an epizootic cough, hoppengarten cough or Newmarket cough; the cause was unknown but it was distinguished from the disease which was then incorrectly being called 'horse influenza'. This is a striking example of how incorrect nomenclature can delay the advance of knowledge. I do not know whether or not this confusion of names existed in Sweden, but when there was an outbreak of epizootic cough in horses in that country in 1955, L. Heller and colleagues thought it worthwhile examining sera of convalescent horses for antibodies against human influenza virus and they obtained positive results. The same disease spread to Czechoslovakia and there Bela Tumova and her colleagues isolated from horses a virus belonging to the influenza A family of viruses. This work was soon confirmed in many countries and it is now well-known that epidemics of respiratory disease in horses are commonly due to equine subtypes of influenza A virus.

Also in 1955 an even more important breakthrough in research on influenza in animals occurred, but in quite a different way. For some years the anatomy of the virus of fowl plague had been known to resemble that of the influenza virus and W. Schäfer in Germany, a research scientist interested in fundamental studies on viruses, discovered that it is in fact a member of the influenza A family of viruses. Fowl plague is a highly lethal disease of chickens bearing no resemblance to influenza clinically and from that point of view no-one could have guessed its virus had any relationship to human influenza A virus. The disease was first described in Italy in 1878 and later was reported in many countries. The causal microbe was shown to be filtrable by two Italians, Centenni and Savonuzzi, in 1901 when only three other filter-passing viruses were known – those causing foot-and-mouth disease of cattle, mosaic disease of tobacco plants, and African horse sickness. The new agent attracted much interest as it was a more convenient model for research into the nature of filter-passers than those previously known. Looking back with our present knowledge we can give the fowl plague virus pride of place as the first influenza virus ever isolated, though it was not recognized as such until much later.

In 1956 two further viruses belonging to the influenza A family were isolated from animals – each a new sub-type – one from ducks in England and one from ducks in Czechoslovakia.

The years 1955–56 opened a new era in studies on the natural history – the ecology – of the influenza virus, although at the time only a few people realized the implications of the discoveries.

OPENING THE PANDORA'S BOX

There was one person who did see the implications of these researches and was in a position to take appro-

priate action, namely Martin Kaplan who was in
charge of the veterinary public health programme of
the World Health Organization (WHO). Kaplan
sought the moral support of Christopher Andrewes and
MacFarlane Burnet and organized a world-wide survey
of horses and pigs for antibodies against influenza. This
was undertaken about the time of the pandemic of
Asian influenza. No antibodies were found against the
Asian virus but in many countries there were antibodies
against the Prague equine influenza virus. Swine influenza was found to have persisted in the U.S.A. and
there was also evidence of it in Czechoslovakia. The
most important consequence of this survey was that it
led to the recruitment of a small group of highly moti-
vated virologists who continued to collaborate with
WHO in the study of influenza viruses in animals. The
programme soon gathered momentum and at yearly
intervals this group of enthusiasts met in Geneva to
review information from all sources and stimulate
interest in the subject. Before long it became apparent
that a Pandora's box had been opened: many subtypes
of the influenza A family of viruses were discovered in
a variety of domestic and wild species.

Swine were found to be infected in many parts of
North America, and also in Hawaii, with a virus that
was the same as, or very like, the one originally discovered by Shope. In 1961 a similar virus was isolated
in Czechoslovakia.

Horses in many countries were found to suffer outbreaks of a coughing disease from which an influenza
virus could be isolated. In 1963 a new equine subtype
suddenly appeared in Miami as though from nowhere
and it behaved just as new subtypes do in man – it swept
across North America and later Europe causing a high

incidence of equine disease. Laboratory tests on horse sera did not reveal any instances of natural infection of horses by human strains.

Some *dogs* were found by Florence Lief of Philadelphia to have antibody to human strains indicating past infections. It seems that human strains occasionally infect dogs but there is no evidence that they spread from dog to dog.

However, it was *birds* that provided by far the greatest harvest of new members of the influenza A family of viruses. In 1959 a strain was isolated from chickens in Scotland and then during the 1960s influenza A viruses were isolated from no less than 46 incidents in domestic and wild birds. Twenty strains were isolated from turkeys, 15 from ducks, 4 from domestic quail, 2 from chickens, 2 from pheasants, 1 from partridges, 1 from pigeons, and 1 from terns (*Sterna hirundo*). Most of these isolations were made in the course of poultry diagnostic work at veterinary laboratories in North America, the U.S.S.R., and Europe, and their significance from the point of view of comparative medicine was often not at first realized. The first isolation from wild birds was from terns that were dying in large numbers near Cape Town, South Africa.

Many of these isolates from animals were carefully studied and classified by Helio Pereira and Geoffrey Schild at the World Influenza Centre in London with assistance from Bela Tumova in Prague. They found that they were all influenza A viruses and had immunological relationships with each other and with human influenza viruses. They could be classified into subtypes as shown in Table 3 and described in Chapter 6.

As far as we know, the strains found in birds are not pathogenic for man but the point has not been investi-

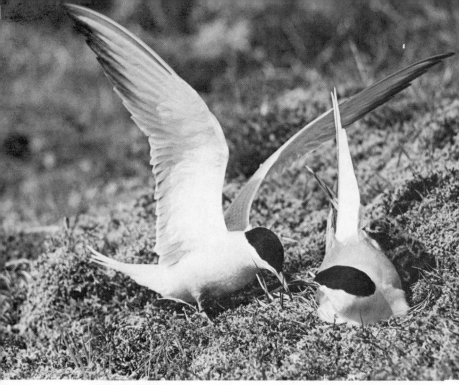

The common tern (Sterna hirundo). *The first influenza virus found in wild birds was isolated from terns in South Africa in 1961.* (Photo Eric Hosking.)

gated experimentally. However, there was one very curious incident which nobody has been able to explain. James Steele, the well-known American veterinary public health worker, was suffering from an attack of hepatitis and one of his research colleagues attempted (unsuccessfully) to isolate the virus of hepatitis from his blood by inoculating it into chick embryos. A virus was isolated which after extensive studies was found to be an avian influenza virus closely resembling that of fowl plague. It is not thought that this virus had anything to do with Steele's hepatitis but the mystery is where did it come from? One possibility was that he had picked it up while travelling abroad. Even if that is correct, why was it in his blood?

Here I have only told the story up to about 1970. Since then investigations on the ecology of influenza virus have expanded and are continuing at an accelerating pace. The latest work, which is producing exciting results with far-reaching implications, will be described in Chapter 9.

THE ILLNESS IN ANIMALS

In pigs the illness caused by the 'classical' swine influenza virus of Shope resembles that in man, as Koen and Aladar observed, except that perhaps it tends to be more severe. The whole herd may be prostrated for several days with the animals showing laboured breathing. However, some mild and even subclinical infections do occur. The mortality may be between one and five per cent but is often less. Since 1970 it has been found that pigs in many countries are commonly infected with the Hong Kong virus, but generally it produces no noticeable ill effects.

In horses the clinical picture is remarkably similar to that in man. If they are not rested during the febrile and convalescent stages, there is a serious risk of respiratory complications, but if horses are well cared for and not returned to work too soon the mortality is very low. Subclinical cases do occur. The equine 2 subtype generally causes a more severe disease than the equine 1 subtype. Killed vaccines give good protection.

Influenza in birds sometimes takes a form similar to that in man, pig, and horse, due allowance being made for signs of disease of such different creatures. However, when discussing birds one must bear in mind that there are many different avian species and many subtypes of virus. There is tremendous variation in susceptibility of different species to a particular subtype, for example the fowl plague virus rapidly kills practically 100 per cent of chickens of all ages; it also causes severe disease in turkeys, but most other species are little affected by it. The influenza virus isolated from wild terns was causing a high mortality in these birds when it was discovered in South Africa. In most outbreaks observed in domestic ducks and quails influenza has taken the form of a respiratory disease. The birds cough, sneeze, and lachrymate and their breathing becomes audible. They may develop sinusitis, swelling of the face, and diarrhoea. There may be signs of involvement of the central nervous system leading to paralysis. Young birds stop growing and adult females stop laying. In turkeys there may be a serious drop in egg production without signs of respiratory disease. We know hardly anything about the effect of the various subtypes on the innumerable species of wild birds, but in a number of cases viruses have been isolated from birds that appeared perfectly normal.

THE HONG KONG VIRUS IN ANIMALS

No authenticated instances of infection of animals with human influenza virus came to light during the era of the Asian subtype and again there was a tendency to believe that generally influenza viruses did not cross from one host species to another, each subtype having an affinity for only one species. But these views had to be revised after the arrival of the Hong Kong subtype in 1968. In 1969, that virus was isolated from pigs in

Taiwan by W. D. Kundin and associates and subsequent investigations showed that in many countries pigs were infected at the same time as the people. However, the strange thing is that the pigs do not become ill when infected with this virus. The next unexpected report was that chickens developed a respiratory disease due to infection with the Hong Kong virus in the Kamchatka peninsula in the far east of the U.S.S.R. Nowhere else in the world had there been reports of infection of chickens with the Hong Kong virus and several deliberate attempts to infect chickens with it had failed. Consequently the report from Russia met with some scepticism in other countries and it was thought there may have been an accidental contamination in the laboratory there, for it is well known that laboratory 'pick-ups' of influenza virus do sometimes occur. Therefore the strain from Kamchatka was inoculated into chickens under experimental conditions in other countries in parallel with a human strain. In all three centres where this experiment was done the chickens inoculated with the Kamchatka strain developed respiratory disease while the others did not.

Shortly afterwards D. K. Lvov, A. Slepuskin, and their Russian colleagues announced that they had isolated a Hong Kong-like virus from a sick calf at Dushanbe, Tadzhik, a town in the Palmirs high up on 'the roof of the world', as this part of south-east Russia is called. Again this report conflicted with experience in other countries where no evidence could be obtained of influenza infecting cattle despite a number of investigations. Therefore the Dushanbe virus was tested in calves in other countries in parallel with a human strain of Hong Kong virus. Just as had happened with the chickens, the Russian virus produced severe respiratory disease in the inoculated calves whereas the human strain had no effect.

Why was it that only in two out of the way corners of the world the Hong Kong virus became adapted to new species? We cannot even guess the answer, but these significant episodes are highly salutary in reminding us yet again that with influenza there are no rules; experience during one period or in one part of the world is only a poor indicator of what to expect at other times and places.

There has been another episode with the Hong Kong virus that has also been instructive. D. O. Johnsen and colleagues in Bangkok inoculated the virus into several gibbons in a colony of 100 of these apes. The inoculated animals did not become ill although virus was recovered from their noses some days later, which showed they had developed a symptomless infection. The strange thing was that between two and three weeks after the inoculations were made thirty-six of the gibbons that had not been inoculated became ill with influenza and four died. The most likely interpretation of these events is that the elapse of some time, during which probably several animal to animal transmissions occurred, was necessary for the virus to become adapted to gibbons. Presumably something of this sort had occurred in the chickens in Kamchatka and the calves in Dushanbe.

The Russians also isolated Hong Kong virus from a dog in Vladivostock. They have also reported finding antibody to Hong Kong virus in fur seals and in mink, but there has been little experience so far with the technicalities of examining sera from these species, so it is too soon to say definitely that these animals had been infected with Hong Kong influenza.

A group of twenty baboons were sent from Nairobi, Kenya, to the Southwest Foundation for Research & Education in San Antonio, Texas, in 1974. Hong Kong virus was found to be circulating among these animals though it produced no signs of illness.

There have also been two isolations of Hong Kong virus from sea birds, one off the coast of Norway and one at the mouth of the Pechora river in northern Russia.

These episodes, where the Hong Kong virus had infected species other than man, show that this human influenza virus has a much wider potential host range than the human influenza viruses prevailing during the thirty-five years between the original isolation in 1933 and the appearance of the Hong Kong virus in 1968. In the light of these findings we must look upon historical reports of influenza in animals with a much more open mind than we have been accustomed to. For example, perhaps we should not dismiss the report that when Charlemagne's army was afflicted with influenza in A.D. 876 the same disease attacked the dogs and the birds. One thing is crystal clear, influenza can no longer be regarded as exclusively or even primarily a human disease.

6

The versatile virus

In Chapter 1 I explained very briefly that there are many different influenza viruses. There are three *types*, A, B, and C, that are not related to one another as judged by the immunity each produces after an attack or vaccination; type A has many *subtypes* and within each subtype there are *variants*. In this chapter I shall explain the nature of the differences between strains as revealed by research on the structure and composition of the virus particles. This knowledge enables us to understand the epidemic behaviour of the disease and provides a sound basis for combating the disease by vaccination and possibly other means.

The anatomy of all influenza viruses is the same. The virus is usually roughly spherical and about 1/10 000 millimetre in diameter, but the shape varies. To compare this size with something familiar, one can say that a clump of viruses the size of an ordinary pinhead would contain about a million million viruses. The surface of the virus is covered with spikes as shown in the photograph taken with the electron microscope, and in the diagrammatic sketch. The spikes on the outside are of two kinds, called haemagglutinin (because it is responsible for clumping or agglutinating red blood cells) and the neuraminidase, which is an enzyme. They

68

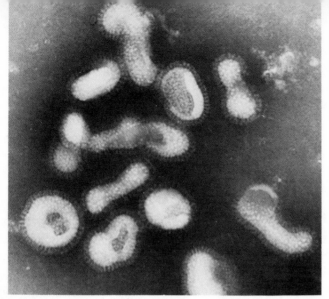

Photograph of influenza viruses magnified about 200 000 times by the electron microscope. (Photo by courtesy of Dr H. P. Chu.)

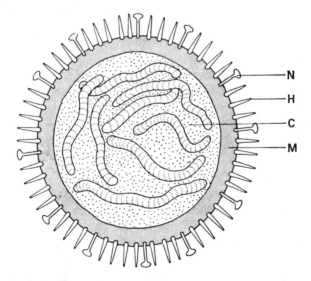

Diagram of a section through influenza virus.
N = Neuraminidase,   H = Haemagglutinin,
C = Core containing genes and protein,   *M = Membrane*

are attached to a membrane or envelope enclosing the core. The core consists of the genetic material of the virus, called ribonucleic acid or RNA for short, together with some supporting protein. An unusual feature of the influenza virus as compared to other viruses is that the RNA is in eight separate pieces, each being a single genetic unit or gene; this has far-reaching consequences as we shall see presently.

The proteins of the virus against which a person or animal produces antibodies when he becomes immune are called antigens. It is the antigens in living viruses and in vaccines that stimulate production of immunity. Influenza virus has four kinds of antigen, the most important ones being the two spikes, the haemagglutinin and the neuraminidase, H and N for short. They are the ones against which protective antibodies are produced. The other two antigens are in the core; they also stimulate the body to produce antibodies but those antibodies do not protect against subsequent infection.

The core antigens and their corresponding antibodies are identical in all subtypes and variants of influenza type A virus. Indeed they are used as the criterion by which to identify a virus as influenza A. The fundamental difference between the type A virus and the type B virus is that there is no relationship whatsoever between any of their antigens and therefore no cross immunity. A person may suffer attacks with both types of virus within a short period of time.

It is the H and N antigens of type A that are of greatest significance for understanding the epidemiological behaviour of influenza. There are many different subtypes of influenza A and each has H and/or N antigens that are quite distinctive immunologically and biochemically. When the new pandemic subtype 'Asian' arose in 1957 it was found that its H and N antigens were both completely different from those of the influenza A viruses that had previously been around and consequently people had no immunity to them. When the new pandemic subtype 'Hong Kong' arose in 1968 it was found to have a new H antigen but the old N antigen. These changes are referred to as antigenic 'shift'. We know no other virus that can change in this way.

There is still another way in which influenza A viruses vary from time to time. The immunological character of the H and N antigens may change slightly every year or so thereby producing variants. These gradual, comparatively-minor variations are referred to as antigenic 'drift', so called because they are believed to be analogous to the phenomenon known as 'genetic drift' in plants and animals.

A change described as a shift is qualitative, whereas one described as a drift is quantitative. It may help explain this if I draw an analogy between antigens and colours. When an H (or N) antigen is quite different from others due to shift, it is as though it is a different colour. When the antigen is a variant due to drift, it is as though it is a different shade of the same colour.

There is usually some degree of cross immunity between the variant strains resulting from drift, though occasionally the drift is rather large and then the new variants are able to infect people immune to the original strain and so produce an outbreak. Influenza B virus is also subject to antigenic drift, but shift has not been observed.

If the reader is to comprehend the epidemiological behaviour and the natural history of influenza it is essential for him or her to keep in mind these characteristics of the virus, so I shall recapitulate. New *subtypes* are produced by *shift* in the H or N antigens and give rise to *pandemics*; new *variants* are the result of *drift* in the H or N antigens and give rise to '*ordinary*' *epidemics* or *localized outbreaks*. Shift and drift both occur in type A virus but only drift with type B.

Some subtypes have been found only in man, some only in horses, some only in birds, and some occur in more than one species. The ability of a virus to infect a particular species is called its 'host affinity'. In biology a virus disease is regarded as an example of parasitism – the virus is the parasite and the animal infected is called the host. At present we do not know what mechanisms determine the host affinity of a strain and the only way we have of finding out is by doing the biological experiment – inoculating the viruses into animals or people.

REPRODUCTION

In order to understand how the influenza virus can change in these ways we must consider how it reproduces. Like all viruses it can multiply only inside living, susceptible cells where it makes use of the cells' chemical workshop and steals the necessary components. First the virus attaches itself to the surface of a susceptible cell, say one of those lining the respiratory tract, by means of its haemagglutinin spikes, and then the cell engulfs it. Once inside the cell, the membrane is shed, releasing the genes, which then make many replicas of themselves. The newly formed genes assemble in sets of eight to make new virus cores. Finally the cores acquire new envelopes and spikes, borrowing some of the constituents of the cell wall. In a matter of hours after entering a cell one virus particle gives rise to as many as 1000 offspring, a new generation of virus particles, which escape from the cell and look for new cells to parasitize.

Antigenic drift is due to mutations in the genes coding for the antigens. These occur during reproduction just as with higher organisms, followed by selective survival of the fittest. For readers not familiar with these biological concepts, let me explain. Mutations are slight chemical changes in the nucleic acid that occur occasionally accidentally during the process of self-copying of the genetic material. When one of these random changes results in a virus particle being less susceptible to the pattern of antibody prevalent in the community, it is better able to survive and multiply than its fellows and therefore outgrows and displaces them. This is exactly analogous to insect pests becoming resistant to insecticides by a similar mechanism.

Antigenic shift was at one time also thought to be due to genetic mutation, but this view has been largely abandoned for reasons set out in Chapter 7. It is now thought that one way by which shift may occur is by the hybridization of two different subtypes. It is possible in the laboratory to arrange for two different subtypes of influenza A virus to infect the same cell. Since the genes of each parent strain are not linked together, they multiply separately and when they assemble into sets of eight to form new cores some of the sets are made up of a mixture of genes from the two parent strains, as though a pack of cards had been shuffled and new hands dealt. This is a primitive form of sexual reproduction. The virus resulting from the mixing of the genes is a hybrid with a new assortment, or combination, of the characteristics of the parents and it breeds true for very many generations. Many viruses are able to produce hybrids

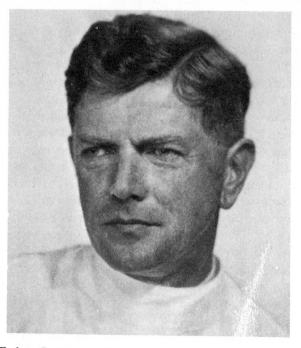

MacFarlane Burnet who discovered that strains of influenza virus can crossbreed and produce stable hybrids.

but influenza strains can crossbreed much more readily than other viruses because the genes are separate.

A FAMILY OF VIRUSES

Let us now relate this knowledge to the pandemics and major outbreaks that have occurred within the last forty years. The viruses isolated up until 1957 all belonged to the same subtype, although gradually quite a lot of

changes occurred over the years by the process of antigenic drift. The H and N antigens of the pre-1957 subtype are designated H1 and N1. (The H antigen of
strains isolated between 1933 and 1946 used to be
designated Ho.) The new pandemic subtype that
appeared in 1957 is designated H2N2, and the Hong
Kong subtype of 1968 is designated H3N2.

Table 3 lists all the subtypes of influenza A known at
present, showing where and when they were first isolated
and their H and N antigens. The antigens from bird
strains are given the prefix av and those from horses eq;
it should be noted that where there is no prefix the
antigens were first recognized in human strains.

The first point to note about the data in Table 3 is
that twenty-three subtypes have been discovered so far,
three from man, two from horses, and eighteen from
birds, that is, six times as many from birds as from man,
despite the fact that much more research has been done
on influenza in man. The second highly significant point
shown in the table is that the antigens in the human subtypes, or antigens related to them, have all been found
in avian subtypes. Thus the N1 of human strains occurs
in chicken/Rostock/1934, in chicken/Scotland/1959, and
in duck/Germany/1968; likewise N2 occurs in turkey/
Massachusetts/1965 and in duck/Italy/1966. The H1
antigen has a relative in chicken/Scotland/1959, and
tern/South Africa/1961; H2 occurs in duck/Germany/
1973; H3 is related to the H antigens of turkey/Canada/
1963 and duck/Ukraine/1963 (also incidentally to
equine 2/Miami/1963). All subtypes are interrelated
like the strands of a spider's web.

The far-reaching implications of the existence of this
large family of influenza A viruses are discussed in
Chapter 7 on the Birth of Pandemics.

Table 3

Subtypes of influenza A

Host	First isolated	N antigen	H antigen (related to)
man	1933 London[1]	1	1
man	1957 Asia	2	2
man	1968 Hong Kong	2	3
swine	1930 Iowa	1	1
horse	1956 Prague	eq1	eq1 (av1)
horse	1963 Miami	eq2	eq2 (3)
chicken	1927 Indonesia[2]	eq1	av1 (eq1)
chicken	1934 Rostock[2]	1	av1 (eq1)
chicken	1949 Germany[2]	eq1	av2
duck	1956 England	av1	av3
duck	1956 Czechoslovakia	av1	av4
chicken	1959 Scotland	1	av5 (1)
tern	1961 South Africa	av2	av5 (1)
turkey	1963 Canada	eq2	av6 (3)
duck	1963 Ukraine	eq2	av7 (3, eq2)
turkey	1963 England	av3	av1 (eq1)
turkey	1965 Massachusetts	2	av6
quail	1965 Italy	eq2	av2
duck	1966 Italy	2	av2
duck	1968 Germany	1	av6
turkey	1968 Ontario	av4	av8
shearwater	1971 Queensland	av5	av6
duck	1973 Germany	av2	2
duck	1974 Tennessee	av6	av3

eq = equine   av = avian

[1] The subtype in man up until 1947 was designated Ho, but recent research indicates that all isolates from man and swine up to 1957 belong to the same subtype which should be designated H1.

[2] These three strains were identified as influenza only after 1955.

LIFE SPAN OF SUBTYPES AND SEROLOGICAL ARCHAEOLOGY

According to our present concepts, the life span of a sub-type affecting man is only from one pandemic to the next. Each subtype causes first a pandemic and then every one to three years epidemics, usually of less importance, which are made possible by antigenic drift. One of the most extraordinary features of the natural history of this remarkable virus is that when a new sub-type arrives it annihilates the old one from the face of the Earth. Each generation of viruses ousts the previous generation and only one human subtype – and usually only one variant of it – exists at any one time. We know of no other virus that behaves in this way; there are many viruses that have subtypes and variants which continue to exist side by side.

Owing to its antigenic novelty, each new subtype or variant is successful in infecting a large proportion of the world's population. This success is detrimental for the survival of the old strain for two reasons: it provokes non-specific reactions against influenza viruses in general by mechanisms such as production of interferon (see page 100), and it may stimulate widespread immun-ity against the old strain (as well as against itself) as a result of the phenomenon known as 'original antigenic sin'. The first time a person is infected with influenza, that particular strain of virus leaves a life-long imprint on the patient's antibody-forming tissues. Every time he gets influenza again he has a recall of antibody to the first strain of influenza virus he encountered, as well as developing antibody to the recent virus infection. The colourful term 'original antigenic sin' was coined by Thomas Francis who discovered this aspect of immunity to influenza.

Here, as in some other parts of this book, I have tended to oversimplify the situation so that a reader new to the subject can easily grasp the main theme. However, I must explain that when a new variant arises it is not always successful in establishing itself throughout the world. There have been several instances where a new variant has been successful for a few months in one region and has died out. Occasionally two variants exist at the same time, and co-exist in many parts of the world for several months before one asserts its supremacy. The one that prevails is usually that with antigens against which the community at large has the lowest level of antibody. We do not yet fully understand why a new strain of influenza virus completely replaces the old one.

We are able to obtain some indication of the nature of past pandemic strains in terms of H antigens by studies known as serological archaeology, that is, by examining the sera of people of different ages for antibodies against the various antigens. Old people still have measurable antibody against strains that infected them as children but have since disappeared and this can be boosted by natural infection or vaccination with present day vaccines. People who were born before the 1918 pandemic have antibodies against swine influenza, which is a variant of H_1N_1. This confirms Shope's contention that the swine virus, which is still circulating in pigs, is a descendant of the virus that caused the 1918 pandemic. Apparently it, or a variant of it, continued to circulate throughout the world for several years because a recent world-wide survey has shown that most people over 50 years of age have antibody to it. Hardly any younger people do, so it must have been displaced in the late 1920s.

People born before 1900 were found to have antibodies against the H antigen of Hong Kong virus (H3) and against that of equine 2 virus (Heq2), these two being related to each other. People born before 1889 were found to have antibodies against the Asian virus (H2N2). The sera of these old people were of course collected before the Asian or Hong Kong epidemics. Therefore it appears that the pandemic of 1889–90 was caused by a subtype with H2 antigens and that around 1900 there was a virus that had H3 antigens.

Another form of archaeology has been attempted in order to study the virus which caused the 1918–19 pandemic. The influenza virus survives for long periods at temperatures below freezing, so it was thought that it might be possible to isolate the virus from the lungs of people who died during the pandemic and were buried in the permafrost in Alaska. In 1951 Albert McKee and his colleagues from the State University of Iowa exhumed some bodies but attempts to isolate a virus failed. Since then more refined techniques for detecting a virus have been developed even when it is no longer viable, so perhaps some further investigations along these lines would yield results of value. However, even the remote possibility of reviving the 1918 virus must be regarded with apprehension and the strictest precautions would need to be taken to avoid any possibility of this terrible pathogen getting loose again.

7

The birth of pandemics

The paramount problem of influenza is how pandemics arise. It is generally agreed that they are the result of the sudden appearance of a new subtype of influenza virus type A but the mystery is, where does the new virus come from or how is it created? The concept of spontaneous generation was of course proved untenable over a century ago and we must seek an explanation consistent with current biological beliefs. Three theories have been put forward: (1) a large genetic mutation of the old subtype, (2) adaptation of an animal virus to man, and (3) hybridization between the old subtype and an animal virus. I shall refer to these as the *mutation*, the *adaptation*, and the *hybridization* theories.

The mutation theory
When in the 1930s and 1940s it was found that there were many variants of the influenza type A virus, it was generally accepted that they arose by genetic mutation from the old strains which they replaced, and this has never been disputed so far as variants are concerned. In 1946, a very large change in the H antigen took place and for some years this was regarded as a shift, introducing a new subtype, but the distinction between drift and shift was not quite so simple as was at first envisaged

and recently more refined analysis of the antigens had led to the view that the 1947 innovation should be regarded as a large drift. In 1957 the Asian virus was acclaimed by all as undoubtedly representing a shift to a new subtype because its H and N antigens were quite unrelated to those of its predecessor. However, the theory that all changes in the virus are due to mutation persisted for some years in many people's minds and they applied it to unquestionable shifts as well as drifts. These adherents to the mutation theory postulated that the virus' genetic make-up had a spectrum of potential antigens which replaced each other in turn, thus as one disappeared in the shift process, former antigens re-emerged. This theory of recycling of antigens was put forward to explain the observations of serological archaeology mentioned in Chapter 6.

However, during the 1960s more and more influenza viruses were isolated from animals and furthermore all the antigens of human strains were found to have their counterparts in animal strains and this fact could not be fitted into the theory of the recycling of the human antigens by mutation. Then in 1971 Graeme Laver, working at the John Curtin School of Medicine, Canberra, Australia, showed by critical biochemical analysis that the H antigens in the viruses circulating just before and just after the start of the Hong Kong (1968) pandemic were quite different from each other chemically as well as immunologically. Furthermore, a search revealed no intermediate or 'bridging' strains such as one would expect if there had been a series of stepwise mutations. It is difficult to believe that such a large jump could occur by genetic mutation. Then similar analyses were done on strains isolated just before and after the start of the Asian (1957) pandemic. Again the biochemical differences as well as the immunological differences were very large and no bridging strains could be found. Besides on that occasion both the H and N antigens changed. Most virologists cannot believe that a change of that magnitude could occur by mutation.

Another difficulty with the mutation theory is that a mutant would be more likely to emerge in the centres of greatest population and when seasonal conditions are most favourable to the spread of the disease, but in fact the very opposite is true. All the information we have points to new subtypes arising away from the main centres of population and often at times of the year when the disease is not very prevalent.

In the light of all the evidence I believe that the mutation theory is no longer tenable as an explanation of the source of new subtypes (except in evolutionary terms, as discussed later) but there are still a few virologists who have not abandoned it.

The adaptation theory
The adaptation theory is that a strain previously confined to some species of animal succeeds in jumping the species barrier, that is, acquires the capability to infect man, probably undergoing some mutation in the factors that determine its host affinity but not its antigenic make-up. This idea of interspecies transfer, or something like it, has roots in history, as we saw in Chapter 5. However, for some years after the isolation of the first influenza virus from man in 1933, it was generally thought that influenza was primarily, if not exclusively, a human disease, the sole exception being swine influenza.

The whole picture has changed dramatically over the last twenty years. Not only have many influenza viruses been isolated from animals but in a number of instances virus has transferred from one species to another, from man to an animal under natural conditions. For example the 1918 pandemic virus and the Hong Kong virus transferred to pigs and the Hong Kong virus transferred to chickens in Kamchatka, U.S.S.R. In addition there have been two reports of isolation of the Hong Kong virus from wild seabirds; one can only speculate whether they caught it from man or whether the birds were its original host from which it spread to man in 1968. During epidemics of influenza in horses over the last twenty years there were several reports from the field that people in the stables caught influenza but when specimens from these cases were examined in the laboratory only in one instance was it possible to confirm infection of man with the equine virus. However, when human volunteers were deliberately inoculated with equine virus they did develop influenza, as also did horses inoculated with human strains of the Hong Kong virus. Very few experiments have been done to test the infectivity of avian subtypes for mammals, but three strains inoculated into ferrets were able to set up infection and produce symptoms.

The general picture one forms as a result of the research over the last twenty years is that each subtype of influenza A virus has a host species to which it is best adapted but that host affinity is not a fixed characteristic and occasionally under favourable conditions a virus can jump the species barrier and become adapted to a new host species. This view is supported by general experience in the laboratory which shows that influenza is a malleable virus in many respects and is amenable to being adapted to laboratory animals.

A special application of the adaptation theory is that a

human strain passes to an animal species and remains
there for a period of years after which it emerges again
and infects man. Richard Shope suggested forty years
ago that an animal species may function as a repository
for a human strain. The much publicized outbreak of
swine influenza in Fort Dix, New Jersey in January 1976
seems to fulfil Shope's prediction. At the time I am
writing it is impossible to say whether this event will
lead to a pandemic but the risk has been judged sufficiently great for the U.S. Government to take the unprecedented step of appropriating $100M to make vaccine
for the entire population.

The hybridization theory

The hybridization theory is that cross-breeding occurs
between a human strain and an animal strain, the offspring virus inheriting its ability to infect man – its host
affinity for man – from the human parent strain and its
H and/or N antigens from the animal parent strain. The
basis for this theory has already been expounded in
Chapter 6, where the genetic mechanism of virus
hybridization was explained.

In the early 1970s Robert Webster and C. H.
Campbell carried out some crucial experiments to test
the hybridization theory. The work was done under
strict isolation at the Plum Island Animal Disease
Laboratories, Long Island, New York. Using pigs,
turkeys, and chickens, and three influenza subtypes that
were pathogenic for one or other of these species, they
mimicked events that could occur naturally by inoculating the animals with two viruses at the same time. It
is unnecessary to describe here the details of these elegant
experiments, but the result was that hybrid viruses
emerged that spread among in-contact animals thus

creating artificially a 'minipandemic'. The new hybrids were stable and would have been capable of causing an epidemic in animals if they had not been confined under rigid security.

In another experiment Webster mixed pigs together after infecting some with Hong Kong virus and some with classical swine influenza, while some were left uninoculated. Within a week a hybrid virus appeared.

These experiments on the production of hybrids in animals finally convinced the sceptics that at least theoretically it is quite feasible for human pandemics to arise in this way. The only possible argument remaining is whether this does actually occur in nature.

It has been known for several years that 'classical' swine influenza, a descendant of the Spanish influenza of 1918, and the Hong Kong virus have both been circulating in pigs in the U.S.A. and several virologists have been watching out for hybrids. Possibly the virus isolated from soldiers at Fort Dix in January 1976 was such a hybrid, inheriting its affinity for man from the Hong Kong parent and its antigenic characters from the swine parent. Alternatively this may have been an example of the virus re-adapting to man without hybridization. The virus now found in swine is not the same as the 1918 virus; it is a distant descendant. During its 58 years sojourn in pigs it has changed in many respects including its affinity and virulence for man. There is no way of knowing whether or not it is capable of regaining the characteristics it had in 1918; one can only say that so far it has not although it has had plenty of opportunity.

We have been concentrating on the human pandemics but both the adaptation and hybridization theories apply equally well to the origin of pandemics in domestic animals. As an example of adaptation there is the case just mentioned of Spanish influenza passing to pigs in 1918 and becoming so well adapted to that species that it has persisted ever since in the U.S.A. although it died out in Europe. Another incident that could be due to either adaptation or hybridization, but probably the latter, was the sudden appearance of a new equine subtype in Miami, Florida in 1963. Despite searching investigations it was not possible to find any trace of it having been introduced from somewhere else. No horse sera collected before the equine 2 outbreak started had antibodies against it. Later it was shown that the H and the N antigens of equine 2 occurred in some avian strains though not both together in the same strain. We do not know when the equine 1 subtype first appeared in horses. It was isolated in Prague in 1956 but old specimens of sera collected long before then were found to contain antibodies to that virus, showing it had been a cause of influenza in horses at least since 1948. Recently it has been found that the antigens of the equine 1 virus are very similar to those of fowl plague, which strongly suggests that this was a case of an avian virus adapting to horses at some unknown time in the past.

Both the adaptation and the hybridization theories fit all the facts we know at present much better than the mutation theory, so it is reasonable to believe that either process may enable the virus to transfer occasionally from animal to man, from man to animal and from one species of animal to another.

We must consider how these theories relate to the historical accounts of influenza occurring at the same time in people and animals. As I have said in Chapter 5, probably some but not all these incidents can be dismissed as mere coincidences. When there were so many horses in the cities and towns and practically all transport depended on them, an outbreak of equine influenza brought business and social life almost to a standstill, causing disruption that is difficult for us to imagine now. Such events obviously made a great impression on people and if influenza occurred in the people about the same time it would be natural to assume there was a causal connection. One gets the impression from reading the reports that they refer not to the start of new pandemics but to outbreaks between pandemics or localized events during the course of a pandemic. The most likely explanation seems to me to be that some of the strains of influenza in the past had a host affinity that was not restricted to one species. We must bear in mind that different subtypes behave in different ways in many respects and our limited experience since the first influenza viruses were isolated only forty-five years ago does not justify our assuming that influenza viruses that prevailed in previous centuries necessarily behaved in just the same way. We have seen how the behaviour of the Hong Kong virus has made us revise some of the ideas formed from experience with the previous human subtypes.

Finally we must consider the rather numerous stories that influenza appeared in horses before it attacked the people. Assuming that in at least some of these incidents the same virus did in fact affect first the animals and then the people, the only explanation would seem to be that the virus was adapted to horses and some weeks were required for it to adapt to man. Possibly the situation was similar to that we have recently witnessed with the swine influenza affecting men at Fort Dix; that is to say, a pandemic virus transferred from man to a species of domestic animal and after some years re-emerged and transferred back to man. Obviously this is simply speculation but I suggest we should not dismiss the historical accounts but let them alert us to what might happen again some time in the future.

EVOLUTIONARY ORIGIN

Table 3 in Chapter 6 shows that in the family of influenza A viruses there are ten different H antigens and ten different N antigens and each subtype is made up of a different combination of one H and one N antigen. Many of the antigens are shared by two or more subtypes from different host species. The only reasonable explanation of this state of affairs is that interbreeding between subtypes occurs from time to time resulting in the swapping of antigens and probably also new combinations of other characteristics such as host affinities. This is an intellectually satisfying explanation of the origin of new subtypes.

The fact that there are so many more subtypes in birds than in mammals and that all antigens found in mammalian strains have their counterparts in birds suggests that the primeval hosts and the main reservoir of the influenza virus A family of viruses are birds. Mammals are also involved but probably to a lesser extent.

There are some 8500 avian species and the total world bird population has been estimated as being of the order of 100 000 million; furthermore, birds have existed in vast numbers for more than fifty million years whereas man is a comparative newcomer and has only been around about two million years. Until a few thousand years ago, or even less, the human population would not have been large enough to support the continued existence of a parasite like the influenza virus which normally produces only a short-lived type of infection. The influenza virus is a parasite that requires a fairly large and dense population to survive.

In accordance with the current biological belief that all living things have evolved by mutation and selective survival, we must assume that this is how the antigens of influenza virus evolved over millions of years. This does not conflict with the conclusion reached above that mutation is not the mechanism by which new pandemic subtypes arise at intervals of 10 to 50 years. A colleague has suggested that I should mention this point. I hope it does not confuse the reader!

CIRCUMSTANCES THAT FAVOUR INTERSPECIES TRANSFER

Having decided that pandemics probably result from the adaptation of an animal strain to man or the hybridization of a human and an animal strain, let us consider the circumstances that would favour these processes taking place.

With many viruses host affinity is not a fixed characteristic and it is common practice in the laboratory to adapt viruses to new hosts, for example mice, for purposes of experimentation. There are six factors that are known to facilitate this transfer and develop the virus' affinity and virulence for the new host. I have summarized these factors below and indicated how they might apply to the birth of pandemics.

(1) *The susceptible age*
Very young animals are much more susceptible to infection with a foreign virus than are mature animals.

Therefore if a baby breathes the same air as infected animals it might take the infection and become the initial link in a chain of human transmissions.

(2) *Dose of virus*
Massive doses are more likely to set up an initial infection than small doses. Exposure to a large dose would occur when a human being spends a lot of time in a confined space with many infected animals.

(3) *Repeated transmissions*
Usually several transfers ('passages' in laboratory jargon) under favourable conditions are needed to adapt a virus to a new host, often the first one to three being critical. This would be most likely to happen where people are living close together.

(4) *Race or breed*
In any species, including man, some races or genetic groups are more susceptible than others to a particular disease and this has been shown in influenza pandemics where, for example, the Eskimoes proved exceptionally susceptible. Probably some races are more likely than others to become initially infected with an animal strain of influenza which would then become adapted to the human race in general.

(5) *Individual susceptibility*
Susceptibility to any microbe, but especially to foreign ones, varies greatly from one individual to another within the same species and race. Therefore the greater the number of people exposed to animal influenza, the greater the likelihood of the one or more exceptionally

susceptible persons meeting the infection and initiating a series of human infections.

(6) *Lowered resistance*
Normal resistance to infections in general is lowered by stress, malnutrition, certain hormonal states or exposure to cold. The presence of another infectious disease may also reduce resistance.

For hybridization an additional circumstance is necessary:

(7) *Simultaneous presence of a human and an animal strain.* Clearly the process of adaptation can only take place in the human host and therefore the animal virus involved must have initially the capacity to multiply to some extent in human cells. Also hybridization could best take place in man but in this case the animal virus need not necessarily be able to actually multiply in human cells; hybridization could occur provided the animal virus had the capacity to enter the human cells and go through the first stage of replication there. It is conceivable that a hybrid pathogenic for man could result from the two viruses mixing in the animal host, but this seems less likely than when they meet in a human being.

The seven factors listed above fit in well with the observations that pandemics arise more frequently in the hinterland of the Eurasian landmass rather than in big cities. There is probably more intimate association between man and a wide variety of animals in that region than anywhere else in the world. In Mongolia and in parts of eastern-European Russia there are vast numbers of domestic animals, the birdlife is said to be

almost unimaginably rich, and wild animals are plenti-
ful. In many of these areas newborn animals are tended
in the same dwelling as the people live with their
babies. In parts of China it is also common for animals
and people to occupy not only the same house but the
same room and there are vast numbers of ducks and pigs,
two animals known to be commonly infected with
influenza viruses. This close association between man
and animals has been going on in central Asia for seven
thousand years.

The question is sometimes asked, why do not new
pandemic strains arise more frequently than they do?
The main reason for the fairly long intervals between
pandemics may be that any new subtype would have to
compete with the old subtype and a small population of
the new virus would be at a disadvantage so long as the
established virus was able to thrive, that is, to find
enough susceptible people to enable it to keep circulating and producing a fairly high incidence of disease.
As explained in Chapter 6, for reasons which we only
partially understand, it is not possible for two subtypes
to exist together. To put it another way, even if new
potential pandemic strains are frequently being thrown
up they cannot emerge until there is a suitable ecological
niche available due to the old strain fading out because
it has exhausted the supply of people susceptible to it.
When the 'swine'-like virus emerged at Fort Dix in
January 1976 it had to compete with the current
'Victoria/75'. The latter proved the more aggressive
spreader and the 'swine'-like virus disappeared, at least
for the time being.

In addition to these considerations, it must be a rare
event for suitable strains to come together under
conditions appropriate for hybridization and to produce

an offspring that has the many exacting requirements necessary for a successful pandemic strain. Moreover, once such a strain has been generated, it needs favourable conditions to build up a critical number of cases to set off a pandemic. It could easily die out in a small scattered community, especially at the wrong time of the year, without ever reaching a large centre of population. A lighted match will only start a fire if placed where there is plenty of tinder.

8

Towards abolishing influenza

In principle there are three strategic approaches to the prevention of influenza: (1) increase the resistance of people by giving them vaccines or drugs, (2) interfere with the spread of the virus, and (3) stop pandemics emerging, the ultimate solution. Vaccination is the most important at present so let us consider it first.

VACCINATION

Vaccines are of two kinds: those made by killing the virus and purifying the effective antigens and those composed of live virus that has been 'attenuated' or modified. Killed vaccines have to be injected, live vaccines are administered into the nose by drop or spray. At present nearly all vaccines that are widely used are killed vaccines. They are made by growing the virus in developing chick embryos, and until a few years ago they produced unpleasant reactions in some people at the site of injection, due to the presence of chick protein and due to some of the components of the virus. However, today much more refined vaccines are available, that seldom give any unpleasant reaction. The immunity conferred lasts only 6 to 12 months, one

94

influenza season, and it reduces the incidence of the disease between 60 and 80 per cent.

Live virus vaccines have been used more in Russia than elsewhere but some extensive trials have been carried out in the U.S.A. and Australia. For a long time the results were generally inferior to those with killed vaccines but during recent years improved methods of attenuating the virus have been developed and the results obtained have been comparable with those from killed vaccines. The virus is now attenuated by exposing it to substances that cause genetic mutation and then selecting out those mutants that grow only at the comparatively low temperature that prevails in the nose and are not able to grow at the higher temperature of the lungs.

Live virus vaccines have the advantage that they are cheaper (because the dose required is smaller), they confer immediate protection, and they are easier to administer, especially in mass vaccination campaigns. Their main disadvantage is that there may be some risk of causing a mild form of influenza, it requires some time to develop strains with the right degree of attenuation, and there is a remote theoretical risk that they might, under very special circumstances, hybridize with other strains and give rise to a new virulent strain.

The chief problem with vaccination with either a killed or live vaccine is that the protection is mainly against the particular variant(s) of virus from which the vaccine is made and only to a lesser extent against other variants. It may confer virtually no protection against variants that are distantly related and it offers none at all against a different subtype. New variants arise every year or two as a consequence of antigenic drift but these are usually not so different as to render the previous year's vaccine useless. Every few years, however, the drift is so large that the vaccine prepared from the previous year's virus gives very little protection. Every decade or so an antigenic shift occurs and then vaccines made from old virus give no protection against the new subtype.

Whenever a major drift or a shift occurs it presents a difficult problem for the vaccine manufacturers. The new virus has to be isolated, its characteristics studied, and it must be trained to grow prolifically in chick embryos before manufacture can start. Then it takes time to prepare vaccine in quantity and to test it for safety and efficacy. Finally there are the logistics of distribution and administration and even then a few days are required before immunity develops. All this takes many weeks, and even months, by which time the virus may have won the race and infected most of the people. However, there is one favourable aspect, namely that pandemics may also have a lag period, as described in Chapter 4.

Successful vaccination obviously depends on early recognition of the emergence of a virus against which it is necessary to prepare a new vaccine. To meet this situation the World Health Organization has established a world-wide network of nearly a hundred collaborating centres throughout the world. These centres are mostly national laboratories that agree to collaborate with WHO. They maintain a constant surveillance – vigilance – on influenza in their locality, isolating strains of the virus, and examining them. Any unusual virus is sent immediately to one of the two WHO Collaborating Centres for Reference and Research on Influenza which are situated in London, England, and Atlanta, Georgia, U.S.A. The many viruses that are sent to these laboratories are scrutinized by the experts there using standard reagents and methods. This excellent scheme ensures that a new variant or new subtype is quickly spotted and everyone concerned is informed immediately. At the end of each winter, vaccine manufacturers confer with specialists at WHO and the WHO Collaborating Centres for Reference and Research on Influenza and decide what strain or strains of virus should be used in preparing vaccine for the following autumn and winter. If there is more than one variant in circulation, the one chosen for the vaccine is that against which samples of the population in several countries have the lowest level of antibody. This is usually the strain farthest removed antigenically from the strain in circulation the previous winter.

Live virus vaccines take as long or longer to develop and test as do killed vaccines but not such large volumes are required and mass vaccination could be carried out more rapidly and at less cost. It would be possible to vaccinate crowds at specially set up emergency centres or even anywhere people congregate such as railway stations, cinemas, etc. The technology has been developed for mass vaccination of chickens against Newcastle disease (due to a virus not unlike influenza virus) and it is common practice to create a fine mist of vaccine in buildings containing thousands of chickens. However, a possible difficulty with human crowds is that one would need to avoid administering live virus vaccine to people who are abnormally susceptible due to chronic ailments such as bronchitis. These people would have to be singled out for injection with killed vaccine. The practical difficulties of mass vaccination with killed vaccines have been greatly reduced by the invention of jet injectors, which do not require needles.

In Brazil recently, 11 million people were vaccinated against meningitis in $4\frac{1}{2}$ days.

The benefit of vaccination goes further than just protecting the individual. Effective vaccination of a person not only prevents a case of the disease, it also eliminates a link in the chain spreading infection. We know that an epidemic occurs only when a large proportion of the population have no antibody, or only a low level of it, against the invading virus. The virus can only spread widely if a large percentage of the population is susceptible. Therefore, vaccinating a proportion of the population would produce the effect known as 'herd immunity'. We do not know what proportion has to be vaccinated to obtain this effect and no doubt it would vary according to several different factors. A reasonable guess might be somewhere between a half and three-quarters in most circumstances.

If the vaccination were deployed strategically in certain groups, such as school children who often provide the tinder for epidemic flare-ups, the community at large might benefit from modest vaccination campaigns. Thomas Francis suggested in 1967 that mass vaccination of school children might be putting vaccination to the best use and this policy was tested out in 1969. Two similar towns in Michigan were selected, Tecumseh and Adrian. In the former town the school children were immunized whereas in the latter no vaccination programme was undertaken. Shortly afterwards the Hong Kong influenza pandemic arrived and there was considerably less influenza in Tecumseh, not only in the school children but also in adults, especially the 20–30 year age group. The present policy in most countries is to protect the most vulnerable groups – those people in whom the disease is most serious, namely those over 60 and those with chronic lung, heart or kidney complaints or diabetes. Also people who are specially at risk – doctors and hospital staffs – may be given a high priority for vaccination.

The survival of subtypes of influenza in man may be much more precariously balanced than is generally realized. Influenza has a very short incubation period and each person is infective to others for only about a week, though a few people may remain carriers of the virus for longer. Consequently the virus must spread quickly or die out. As we have seen, the last two pandemics did not at first spread well in Europe or America in spite of the fact that the whole population was susceptible. Also we have seen that old subtypes are eliminated entirely when a new subtype arrives. The 1918 pandemic virus set up disease in pigs in the U.S.A., Hungary, and England and probably in other countries but it died out everywhere except in the U.S.A. It may turn out that it is not such a very formidable task to stop pandemics in future when we have improved weapons.

DRUGS

In view of the variability of the immunological·characters of the influenza virus and the consequent difficulty of preparing the appropriate vaccine in advance of an outbreak, and in the light of the success of drugs and antibiotics against bacterial and protozoal diseases, a great amount of research has been directed towards developing drugs that will prevent or cure influenza. When drugs are taken to prevent a disease as distinct from curing it, as for instance against malaria when visiting a known infected area, this is called chemoprophylaxis. Some encouraging results with chemo-prophylaxis against influenza have been obtained with several compounds, the best known being amantadine, which has already been mentioned in connection with the treatment of the illness. This drug has been shown to have some preventive effect against influenza in mice, turkeys, horses, and quails. Trials conducted in human volunteers showed the drug could be used to prevent the disease but it has not been widely used because it has some undesirable side-effects. A related compound, rimantadine, has been developed that is more effective in mice. This drug has been tried out in people living in the same house as patients ill with influenza. In controlled trials it reduced the percentage of those that became infected from 14 to 3.6 per cent. It seems that rimantadine may be useful in special situations but it has to be taken twice a day over the whole period of risk.

In 1957, Alick Isaacs, working at the National Medical Research Institute, London, discovered that when influenza virus infects tissue, the cells produce an antiviral substance which he called interferon. He showed that recovery from influenza is due largely to interferon rather than to antibody. The antiviral action of interferon is not limited to particular subtypes or variants like antibody is. Much research has been devoted to attempting to develop a preparation of interferon that could be used to prevent or treat the disease. The idea is extremely attractive as this is a substance that the body produces naturally for combating the virus and it has none of the objections that there are to most drugs. Unfortunately so far no one has succeeded in overcoming the practical difficulties. More recently it has been discovered that certain relatively simple compounds stimulate the body to produce interferon in the

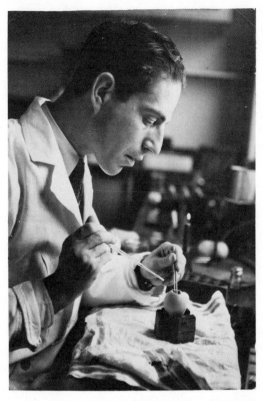

Alick Isaacs examining a chick embryo that had been inoculated with fluid from a patient's throat. He discovered interferon which helps us recover from influenza. (Photo by courtesy WHO.)

same way that the virus does and at one time there were great hopes that anti-influenzal effects could be obtained by administering these so-called interferon inducers. However, again practical trials have given disappointing results with the interferon inducers so far available.

As with vaccination, an effective antiviral drug used on a mass scale and strategically could prevent or stop

I.—8

an epidemic even though not all the people were treated. An obvious advantage over vaccination is that the influenza virus could not circumvent such a barrier by a change of its antigenic make-up, but it might develop drug resistance. A further disadvantage of a drug is that it has to be taken continuously all the time that the virus is about. One day efficient chemoprophylaxis against influenza will be possible but there is no sign yet of a miracle drug that could be used on a mass scale.

PREVENTING THE SPREAD OF VIRUS

Many diseases of domestic animals can be kept in check by quarantine measures but human populations are far too mobile today for quarantine procedures to be feasible.

About thirty years ago there was a spate of research into ways of preventing the spread of airborne infection by creating antiseptic vapours in the air of buildings and by the use of ultraviolet light, which is lethal to the virus. Some chemicals were found to kill the virus in the air when they were sprayed as a fine mist or vapourized but unfortunately there were practical objections of one sort or another to all of them.

Many experiments have been carried out to see how long various viruses can survive in the air under different conditions. One unexpected finding was that they are killed more quickly in the open air than in buildings even when temperature, humidity, and light were held constant. The nature of this open-air factor was not discovered but it is widespread, at least in England. Clearly there is need for more research here and these observations encourage one to hope that a harmless substance will one day be found that can be used to kill the virus in the air in buildings, trains, etc. and stop the spread of influenza.

Another way of approaching this subject is for people to wear a mild antiseptic substance around their neck or on a mask. Thus each person would carry around his own protective aura – something like a lady wearing perfume – and when a group or crowd gathered there would be an appropriate build up of the vapour in the surrounding air. At one time it was customary for people to wear a piece of camphor in a small sack under the front of their shirt when influenza was about. This is an attractive idea but the difficulty is to discover something that is both safe and effective. There was some experimental work done that suggests the method might be feasible. MacFarlane Burnet showed that mice can be protected against virus sprayed into the air by painting the outside of their noses with a dilute solution of iodine.

Ultraviolet light has been used on a limited scale in hospitals and in schools and has been shown to reduce the spread of some infections. However, the present indications are that under most circumstances ultraviolet light is of little value against a widespread airborne infection like influenza.

Since the Middle Ages some people have tried to protect themselves against infections of various sorts by wearing masks. During the 1918–19 pandemic in various countries cotton gauze face masks, as used by surgeons, were worn fairly extensively, sometimes treated with antiseptics. There is no good evidence that they were of any value and it has been shown that they have very little effect in filtering out fine particles from the inspired air. Improved masks have been made of paper but they are not much better. One problem is that air passes around the edges of the mask.

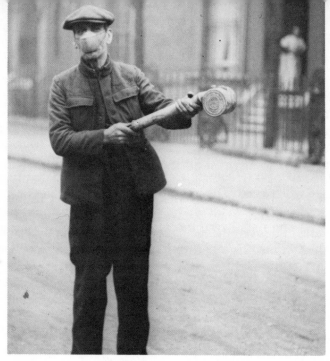

In 1918 buses and sometimes even streets were sprayed with disinfectant in a desperate but futile attempt to stop influenza spreading.
(Photo. RadioTimes Hulton Picture Library)

In many cities in the U.S.A. and elsewhere the police wore masks during the Spanish influenza pandemic for their own protection and to set an example.
(Photo. Radio Times Hulton Picture Library)

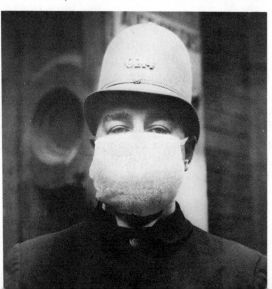

Of course the purpose of masks in surgery is to protect the patient, not the wearer. To protect the wearer one needs an industrial type of mask. Masks have been developed that are quite light and effective in filtering out particulate matter and in certain industries operators wear them all the working day, even sometimes while doing heavy work. The main problem is to get a good fit, to ensure that all the air passes through the filter and none around the edges of the mask. Masks of this type have not been used to any appreciable extent in medicine as they have been thought to be too unpleasant for the wearer.

There is scope for more research on various aspects of air hygiene. Everything that has been learnt so far only reinforces the time-honoured virtues of fresh air and sunshine, avoiding crowded places, and contact with people you know are infective. When people cough and sneeze they should cover their faces with handkerchiefs. Also it helps if people stay at home at the first sign of influenza. The spread of infection could be reduced significantly if people were conscientious about not contaminating their environment – 'coughs and sneezes spread diseases'.

THE ULTIMATE SOLUTION

At the time I am writing, the World Health Organization is on the verge of achieving the eradication of smallpox from the world. Eradication of influenza viruses from their reservoir in wild animals, especially birds, is inconceivable but I believe the time has now come for us to start thinking seriously about the possibility of preventing new human pandemic subtypes emerging. We are still very far from knowing enough to enable us to prepare a programme for such a defence against the disease, but we can now see that if we work along certain lines it might be possible to do something of this sort within a couple of decades. This goal does not seem to me so far off as landing men on the Moon did twenty years before they got there. What I suggest we should do now in order to progress towards that goal is discussed in the next chapter.

9

The continuing quest

RECENT AND CURRENT INVESTIGATIONS IN BIRDS

In Chapter 5 I told the story of the discovery of influenza viruses in birds up to about 1970. Since then new discoveries have followed one another at an exciting pace.

During the 1960s the virus isolations were nearly all from domestic birds, principally turkeys and ducks. In most instances the outbreaks were isolated episodes that could not be traced to previous outbreaks in poultry and it was generally thought that they had originated from wild birds. In a number of surveys antibody to influenza virus was found in wild birds. Sick or dead wild birds are not often found as predators and scavengers quickly remove them and the prospect of finding virus in apparently healthy birds seemed as formidable as looking for the proverbial needle in a haystack. Nevertheless this daunting task was attempted in a number of places, especially in the U.S.S.R. and U.S.A. The procedure was to capture or shoot the birds and take specimens from their windpipes with swabs and to collect blood. Many hundreds of specimens were collected and each processed in the laboratory. A lot of the surveys involving considerable trouble and expense yielded only negative results. For example, WHO assisted in making arrangements with the Peruvian

Government for Robert Webster and Graeme Laver to collect specimens from the birds which exist in vast numbers off the coast of that country. Specimens were taken from 300 birds but not a single one contained either antibody or virus.

Gradually more promising areas and species were found. One of the first successes came from the Great Barrier Reef off the north-east coast of Australia. In 1971, Graeme Laver and J. C. Downie isolated a virus from a shearwater (*Puffinus pacificus*) and it turned out to be a new subtype. In 1972, D. K. Lvov and his colleagues at the Ivanovsky Institute of Virology in Moscow mounted a large-scale operation in several outlying regions, mainly involving migratory birds in the far east of the U.S.S.R., around the Caspian Sea and in the Archangel region in the far north. This programme is continuing and despite having drawn a blank in several surveys they have to date made over 100 isolations from wild ducks, herons, terns, gulls, guillemots, crows, and other species.

Also in 1972 a large programme was launched in the U.S.A. involving a number of virologists, those mainly responsible being Bernard Easterday of Madison, Wisconsin, and Richard Slemons of Washington, D.C. They concentrated on migrating waterfowl which were captured or shot on the Atlantic, Mississippi, and West Coast flyways. This proved to be a rich source of virus and they have made over 100 isolations from ten of the thirty-five species examined. Table 4 gives some details of six of these investigations. It will be seen that in September–October 1974 there were 24 isolations from 494 birds – about 5 per cent.

This remarkably high isolation rate was probably due to a surprising discovery made in 1974 that may

Table 4

Isolation of influenza virus from migrant birds in the U.S.A.

Investigators	Date of collection	Location	Number and type examined	Species yielding virus	Number of isolations
R. D. Slemons & colleagues	Oct.–Dec. 1972	West Coast flyway, California	2000 migrant waterfowl	Pintail, teal, mallard, ruddy shoveller, gadwall	41
A. K. Bahl & colleagues	Sept. 1973	Mississippi flyway, Minnesota	60 migrant waterfowl	Mallard	4
J. K. Rosenberger & colleagues	Nov. 1973	Atlantic flyway, Delaware, and Maryland	159 migrant waterfowl	Mallard, black duck, Canada goose	4
R. G. Webster & colleagues	Nov. 1973– Jan. 1974	Mississippi flyway, Tennessee	829 migrant waterfowl	Ducks	6
B. C. Easterday & colleagues	Sept.–Oct. 1974	Mississippi flyway, Wisconsin	494 migrant waterfowl	Mallard, wigeon, teal	24
B. C. Easterday & colleagues	July–Aug. 1975	Point Barrow, Bering Sea	308 Arctic and other seabirds	Sabine's gull, Arctic tern	2

revolutionize our notions about the ecology of the influenza virus. It was found that the virus can be isolated much more frequently from swabs taken from the cloaca than those taken from the respiratory tract. Remember these were migrating birds that were apparently in good health! Exactly what tissue the virus was multiplying in and how long it usually persists there remains to be found out. This fruitful source of virus is now being investigated in the U.S.S.R. and elsewhere. It is too soon to draw conclusions but it looks as though the real home of the influenza virus may prove to be some non-respiratory tissue of birds from which it is shed in the droppings.

Yet another source of avian influenza virus was stumbled on unexpectedly during the last few years, this time closer to home – in pet birds. In 1971, three strains of influenza virus were isolated from myna birds imported into California and Florida. About that time there were severe outbreaks of Newcastle disease in chickens in California and there was suspicion that the disease had been introduced by cagebirds which had been imported from Thailand. Therefore all imported birds were examined for the Newcastle disease virus and in the process many strains of influenza virus were isolated. In a period of just six months from January to July 1972 Richard Slemons and his colleagues made fifteen isolations from the following birds: myna, finch, fairy bluebird, green weaver, oriole, sunbird, flowerpecker, banded pitta, sharma thrush and hoopoe from Thailand, a parrot from Mexico, and a paradise tanager from Equador.

Many isolations were also made from cagebirds imported into Europe. Between 1970 and 1973 in Britain and in Germany virus was found in a number of cockatoos, parrots, and parakeets, and also in a hornbill. These birds had come from Australia, Africa, South America, and India but it was not possible to determine whether they had picked up the virus in their native land, during transport or after arrival in Europe. Most of them were ill or dead when examined but usually the cause was some condition other than influenza.

In 1975, Henry Chu of the Veterinary School at Cambridge, England, hit on the idea of examining cagebirds that were dead on arrival at London Airport. Large numbers regularly arrive there from many countries and there is often considerable mortality, due mainly to the conditions of transport rather than disease. Chu examined birds from 86 consignments during 1975 and in no less than 28, that is 32 per cent, he isolated influenza virus. Most of the birds were parakeets from India or Pakistan but he also found virus in two lots of finches and two lots of myna birds.

Altogether some hundreds of strains of influenza virus have now been isolated from a wide range of birds in many countries. It is hard to believe that just a few years ago we were ignorant of the situation. One of the first questions asked was what is the relation of these wild bird viruses to the avian subtypes listed in Table 3 on page 76 that were nearly all found originally in domestic poultry? It has been something of a relief to find that most of them belong to the recognized subtypes. It is quite likely that we have not yet captured all the subtypes that exist but it now looks as though the total range will not extend far beyond the present list. It may not be out of the question to produce vaccines against all the antigens. One could ignore the N antigens as the H antigens are sufficient to produce immunity.

QUESTIONS SELDOM ASKED

The main thrust of research on influenza over the last twenty years has been applying modern, sophisticated, technical methods to reveal details of the structure and chemical composition of the virus, the mechanisms whereby it propagates itself, and its interaction with its host in terms of immunology. It has been exciting for both workers and watchers and much knowledge has been gained, but this book is mainly concerned with broad biological aspects of the disease, some of which have not received the attention they merit. My special interest is the ecology of the virus in animals and I shall return to this subject presently, but first I would like to point out some other questions for which we need answers.

What are the mechanisms that determine whether or not a strain of virus can infect a particular host species and the degree of damage it will cause if it does?
Host affinity and virulence are two related characters of the virus that are of crucial importance. They can be manipulated experimentally to some extent and it should be feasible to investigate the underlying mechanisms by modern techniques. Antigenic analysis has so dominated our classification of the strains that other biologically-important characters have been neglected. We should try to find 'markers' by which host affinity and virulence can be determined in the laboratory without recourse to inoculation of animals or human volunteers.

Why is it that even in severe pandemics usually about half the population do not develop the disease?
The indications are that in severe pandemics like that

of 1918 practically everyone becomes infected and develops antibodies against the virus, which means that many people undergo an active infection without becoming ill. A lot is known about specific, acquired immunity but very little about non-specific resistance, although it is of the greatest importance, and if we could learn how to manipulate it our control of infectious diseases might be revolutionized. An associated problem is why does the incidence vary considerably from one group of people to another and from one town to another?

Why does influenza spread well in the winter months but poorly or not at all in the summer, although it spreads in warm weather in the tropics?
We can guess at the nature of some of the seasonal factors that determine the dissemination of the disease, but is there also an as yet undefined 'winter factor' as many writers assert? Perhaps a better understanding of the factors that are unfavourable to influenza in summer would enable us to use them against it in the winter.

If we could crack any of these problems, an entirely new way of combating the disease might be revealed. But they are difficult problems and await someone with a fresh approach and new ideas. Meanwhile ecological studies are opening up new vistas and here we can see a perfectly feasible scheme that urgently needs putting into practice now.

PLOTTING THE COURSE AHEAD

In every country there are public health laboratories that keep a constant watch on infectious diseases of

people and veterinary laboratories with responsibilities
for diseases of domestic animals, but there are hardly
any laboratories whose concern it is to investigate
diseases of wildlife. Therefore special arrangements are
needed to investigate influenza in wild birds and
mammals. As mentioned above, there is a well-
organized programme in the U.S.S.R. and U.S.A., but
in the rest of the world there are only a few isolated
investigators. The World Health Organization has done
much to stimulate and co-ordinate work in this field
with very modest expenditure but so far only the tip of
the iceberg has been revealed. The recent discoveries
have established the importance of this subject and I
believe a greatly expanded programme is now called for.

The following is a brief outline of the programme on
the ecology of influenza virus that I suggest would be
appropriate. It should be organized by some central
body such as the World Health Organization with funds
provided specifically for this work. Collaboration could
be solicited from suitably staffed and equipped laboratories located at strategic points on all continents. These
would form a co-ordinated network of investigation
centres and be linked with the WHO collaborating
centres for human influenza. The investigation centres
would undertake systematic surveys of domestic and
wild animals, paying particular attention to wild birds
since they seem to be the richest source of viruses and
many of them range freely world-wide. Collecting
specimens from wild birds is not such a formidable task
as it may at first appear. Assistance can often be obtained from ornithologists who trap birds to put bands
on their legs for identification; in many countries wild
birds are shot in large numbers and the hunters usually
have no objection to laboratory specimens being col-

lected from the dead birds; in some places scientists studying the epidemiology of insect-borne viruses capture birds as part of their work and they could easily at the same time take specimens for influenza studies; finally many birds are caught for the cagebird trade.

The first objective would be to capture the full range of influenza A subtypes. Their antigens would be studied by specialists at central laboratories and be made available for the preparation of particular vaccines if and when required. It might be feasible to stockpile some vaccine against all the principal haemagglutinin antigens to be used in a fire-brigade type of action as soon as an incipient pandemic is spotted.

The next step would be to investigate the natural and potential range of host affinity and virulence of the various subtypes and strains for domestic birds and mammals, both by contact and by inoculation into the young of the possible new host.

The long term programme would be to study the ecology of influenza viruses found occurring in domestic or wild animals. This would include finding out which species are infected and the epidemiology within each species (the age infection takes place, how long they remain shedders, etc.), any spread between species, the geographic distribution, and seasonal incidence. Particular attention would be given to points of contact and possible transfer of infection from wild to domestic animals. Probably the virus in wild species does not constitute a threat to man until it gets into domestic species where it has the opportunity of extensive and intensive contact with man. Domestic animals could constitute a bridge between wild animals and man.

When the next pandemic arises, an intensive investigation should be carried out in the region where the primary focus occurs in an attempt to trace its origin.

The central organizing body would collect and marshal information from all sources and periodically arrange meetings of specialists to review it and plan the next moves.

When potentially dangerous situations were detected appropriate precautionary measures would need to be considered. For example, the people who come in contact with infected animals might be vaccinated against the appropriate strain of virus. Another possibility would be to combat the infection in domestic animals by such measures as vaccination, changed husbandry methods or eradication of the infection using accepted veterinary hygiene measures. Perhaps imported cage-birds should be quarantined and examined for virus before being sold to the public. These are just tentative suggestions, at this stage it is not possible to foresee where these investigations will lead and what possible lines of action may open up.

SUMMING UP

Influenza is different from all other diseases in fundamental ways that make it refractory to control measures effective against others, therefore new approaches must be sought. Pandemics of the black death, cholera, yellow fever, typhus, and smallpox are things of the past in most parts of the world because their means of transmission have been controlled or there are highly efficient vaccines. But public health procedures do not deter the airborne virus of influenza and vaccines against it have only a limited, temporary effect. Influenza flourishes in the modern world and there is no sign that the position will change significantly unless we can find a radical solution to the problem.

The evidence presented in this book indicates that there is a reasonable hope that world-wide studies on the ecology of the virus may eventually show how influenza pandemics can be prevented. One of my aims has been to draw the attention of those who administer research to the possibilities and opportunities.

Parasites prosper when their hosts become numerous and crowded. The human race has become very numerous and crowded. Huge aggregations of people and a vast air transport system have provided ideal conditions for the spread of the airborne parasite we are concerned with. Influenza pandemics could well become increasingly serious, and there is no known reason why there should not be another catastrophic one like that of 1918 or even worse. The disease known as fowl plague, due to an influenza virus, causes practically 100 per cent mortality in chickens. Influenza is no respector of national or climatic barriers and affects rich and poor countries alike. It is a global plague: a spark in a remote corner of the world could start a fire that scorches us all. But one day man will find out how to tame this versatile virus; the story of discovery is not yet finished.

Milestones

1931   Influenza virus isolated from swine.

1933   Influenza virus isolated from man.

1935   Influenza virus cultivated in chick embryos.

1936   Variants of the (type A) virus found to exist.

1940   Second type (B) of influenza virus isolated.

1941   Haemagglutination (clumping of red blood cells by virus) discovered.

1943   Killed vaccine developed and shown to be effective.

1946   Novel variant 'A prime' emerged, thought at the time to be a new subtype (H_1N_1).

1949   Stable hybrids produced in the laboratory by crossbreeding different strains.

1955   Avian influenza viruses recognized.

1955   Influenza virus isolated from horses.

1957   Neuraminidase identified.

1957   Interferon discovered.

1957   **Asian Pandemic,** new subtype (H_2N_2) emerged.

1961   Influenza virus isolated from wild birds (terns).

1963   Amantadine, the first drug active *in vivo* against influenza.

1968   **Hong Kong Pandemic,** new subtype (H3N2) emerged.

1971   Hybridization demonstrated in live animals.

1972   Influenza virus found to occur frequently in wild birds.

1974   Influenza virus found in cloaca of wild birds.

1976   Swine influenza outbreak at Fort Dix, New Jersey, (January).

Glossary

Antibody specific substance in the blood serum produced by the body to help combat an invading microbe; in the laboratory antibodies react only against the corresponding antigen.

Antigen protein against which the body produces antibody; every microbe has several different kinds of antigen.

Chemoprophylaxis prevention of disease by administration of a drug before infection occurs.

Cloaca sac inside a bird's anus which receives the faeces and urine before they are voided.

Drift antigenic drift; gradual, relatively-minor changes in the antigen(s) of the virus.

Droplet nuclei minute particles remaining in the air after the water has evaporated from droplets emitted from the nose or mouth during sneezing and coughing.

Enzyme a protein able to transform particular substances without being changed itself.

Gene unit of heredity, nucleic acid (RNA or DNA) with a specific composition carrying the code for hereditary characters.

Haemagglutinin (H) one of the two antigens on the

surface of the influenza virus; it is able to attach to cells and it causes clumping (agglutination) of red blood cells in the laboratory.

Host affinity affinity of a virus for a particular host species, the ability of the virus to infect a species of animal (the host).

Hybrid crossbred organism inheriting some characteristics from each of widely different parents.

Interferon defensive substance produced by cells when they are infected by a virus.

Marker characteristic recognizable in the laboratory that helps to identify a particular strain of virus.

Miasma noxious emanation, especially air containing hypothetical disease-causing substances arising from the soil, earth or decomposing organic material.

Mutation acquisition of a new characteristic due to a change in the genetic (hereditary) make-up; genetic mutations are due to slight chemical changes in the nucleic acid that occur occasionally by accident during self-copying of a gene in the course of reproduction.

Neuraminidase (N) one of the two antigens on the surface of the influenza virus; it is an enzyme.

Pandemic very widespread epidemic; with influenza it has come to mean a worldwide epidemic due to a new subtype of the virus.

Serological archaeology study of the antibodies in the serum of people of different ages; old people have antibodies against viruses that infected them in their youth but have since disappeared.

Serology study of antibodies in serum, identification

of antibodies by seeing if they react with particular antigens.

Shift   antigenic shift; sudden complete change of one or more of the antigens of the virus.

Type, Subtype, Variant   terms used in classifying microbes: those belonging to one type, subtype or variant have certain characteristics in common, especially antigens; a subtype is a subdivision of a type and a variant is a subdivision of a subtype.

Virus   minute microbe able to pass through filters that hold back bacteria and too small to be seen with an ordinary microscope; they can reproduce only inside living cells.

Index